Samantha Towle is a *New York Times*, *USA Today*, and *Wall Street Journal* bestselling author. She began her first novel in 2008 while on maternity leave. She completed the manuscript five months later and hasn't stopped writing since.

She is the author of contemporary romances, The Storm Series and The Revved Series, and standalones, *Trouble*, *When I Was Yours*, *The Ending I Want*, *Unsuitable*, *Wardrobe Malfunction*, *Breaking Hollywood*, *Under Her* and *Sacking the Quarterback*, which was written with James Patterson. She has also written paranormal romances, *The Bringer* and The Alexandra Jones Series. All of her books are penned to the tunes of The Killers, Kings of Leon, Adele, The Doors, Oasis, Fleetwood Mac, Lana Del Rey, and more of her favorite musicians.

A native of Hull and a graduate of Salford University, she lives with her husband, Craig, and their son and daughter in East Yorkshire.

Keep up with Samantha and her upcoming releases at **www.samanthatowle.co.uk**, find her on Facebook: **www.facebook.com/samtowlewrites** or follow her on Twitter: **@samtowlewrites**.

By Samantha Towle

Gods Series
Ruin

Standalone
The Bringer
Trouble
When I Was Yours
The Ending I Want
Sacking the Quarterback (with James Patterson)
Unsuitable
Wardrobe Malfunction
Breaking Hollywood

Revved Series
Revved
Revived

Storm Series
The Mighty Storm
Wethering the Storm
Taming the Storm
The Storm

Alexandra Jones Series
First Bitten
Original Sin

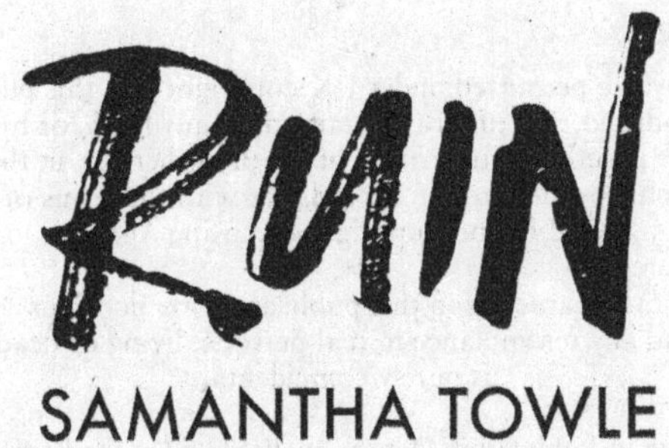

SAMANTHA TOWLE

HEADLINE
ETERNAL

First published in Great Britain in 2018
by HEADLINE ETERNAL
An imprint of HEADLINE PUBLISHING GROUP

4

Cataloguing in Publication Data is available from the British Library

ISBN 978 1 4722 5147 3

Typeset in Sabon LT Std by Jouve (UK), Milton Keynes

Printed and bound in Great Britain
by Clays Ltd, Elcograf S.p.A.

Headline's policy is to use papers that are natural, renewable and recyclable products and made from wood grown in well-managed forests and other controlled sources. The logging and manufacturing processes are expected to conform to the environmental regulations of the country of origin.

HEADLINE PUBLISHING GROUP
An Hachette UK Company
Carmelite House
50 Victoria Embankment
London EC4Y 0DZ

www.headlineeternal.com
www.headline.co.uk
www.hachette.co.uk

RUIN

Prologue

Zeus

THE ARENA IS FULL. Thousands of people are here to watch this fight.

Watch me fight.

This is where I've gotten. The point I've reached in my career.

Everything I've had to do—endure, sacrifice—has brought me to this moment.

I'm waiting in the dressing area with my team, ready to go. TV cameras are with me, ready to follow me to the ring.

It's a big production. My manager, Marcel Duran, likes to make a show out of everything.

I don't give a shit about any of that.

I just want to fight.

It's all I know. All I'm good at.

Twenty-five years old, I'm undefeated. Olympic champion. International Boxing Federation and World Boxing Council world heavyweight champion.

But my opponent, Kaden "The Canadian Devil" Scott, has the World Boxing Organization title, and I want it.

It'll give me three titles.

And I always get what I want.

Then, after this fight, I'm going for the other two titles—World Boxing Association and the International Boxing Organization—held by that fucker Roman Dimitrov.

I get those, and I'll have all five. I'll unify the division.

I'll be the ultimate.

I'd say it'd make me a god, but I already am.

Zeus "The God" Kincaid.

I was born to do this.

And every fucking thing I've lost and had to sacrifice to get here will be worth it.

The hush comes. My heart pounds harder and faster.

I get to my feet.

The cameras move in front of me. I don't focus on them. I can't. I'm already in my head.

Walk to the ring. Fight. Win.

That's all I can think about.

I bounce on my heels. I'm wired. Restless. Pent-up energy that I'm about to expel on the Canadian's face.

The crackle of the microphone echoes throughout the stadium.

Then, the most recognizable voice in the boxing world starts to speak, "Ladies and gentlemen, get on your feet and be upstanding to welcome your champion . . . Zeus . . . 'The God' . . . Kincaid!"

The soft piano beginning of Eminem's "Lose Yourself" starts to hum throughout the stadium.

I always come out to this song.

Because it's what I do when I fight. Lose myself. I forget everything and everyone. Forget my regrets, my mistakes.

I forget *her.*

The beat kicks in, and that's my cue. I start walking. Out of the dressing area. Into the hall toward the tunnel.

White curtains hang in front of me, ready to reveal me.

I don't break stride as they're drawn back by two ring girls dressed in togas.

The tunnel is lined with Grecian pillars. Marcel fucking loves to ham "The God" theme up.

I jog up the steps and into the arena.

The screams are deafening.

People. Lights. Strobes. Pyrotechnics.

I hear and see none of them.

I see one thing.

The ring. And the person waiting in it for me.

My whole being is taut, rigid, focused as I walk toward the ring, flanked by my team.

A quick glance to where I know my family is sitting—my brothers, Ares and Lo, and my sister, Missy—and then I'm up the steps. I slip in between the ropes.

And it's time.

My eyes meet Scott's across the ring.

He looks hard. Empty.

But I'm harder and emptier.

Two rounds, motherfucker, and you're done.

My music fades out, and the announcer starts to speak again, "And here's the moment we've all been waiting for. Our fighters are in the ring, and they are ready. In the blue corner, standing at six feet four inches and weighing in at two hundred forty pounds, the current WBO heavyweight champion of the world . . . 'The Canadian Devil' . . . Kaden Scott!"

There are a few cheers but more boos from the crowd. Not because Scott's an ass. From what I know, he's a decent guy. But he's Canadian, and we're in my home country tonight.

And, of course, I'm better.

"And, in the red corner, standing at six feet six inches and weighing in at two hundred fifty pounds, he is the IBF and WBC world heavyweight champion—twenty and O with twenty knockouts—your homegrown champion . . . 'The God' . . . Zeus Kincaid!"

The crowd roars. I lift my arms in the air, like I've already won. Because, in my mind, I already have.

And he continues, "To the thousands in attendance and the millions watching at home, ladies and gentlemen, from Boardwalk Hall in Atlantic City . . . let's . . . geeet . . . rrrreeeaaady . . . toooo . . . ruuummmble!"

The crowd is cheering.

And I'm ready to fight.

I go to my team. My robe is taken off.

I sit down on the stool.

"You've got this, Zeus." My trainer, Mike, is in front of me, his hands on my shoulders, his face in mine. "You can nail this motherfucker. He's good. But you're better. Three rounds, tops, and he's yours."

"Two," I rumble out before my shield is put in my mouth.

I'm up on my feet. I go to the center of the ring. My team follows.

The referee stands between Scott and me.

I focus on Scott. From hours spent watching tapes of his previous fights, my eyes are on the weaknesses I already know he has.

A fractured cheekbone from a year ago. Cuts easy above his right eye. Nose broken four times.

The referee starts talking, "We went over the rules in the dressing rooms. I want you to keep it clean at all times. Protect yourselves at all times. And what I say, you must obey. Good luck to both of you. Touch gloves. Back to your corners."

We bang gloves. I turn and walk back to my corner.

Mike is in my ear with last-minute directions. "Don't go in fast. Make him come to you. Step back when he swings. Frustrate him. It's his Achilles heel. Scott has no patience."

The bell rings, and I go in, fists up.

We fight. Longer than I expected. He's a tough motherfucker.

We're nine rounds in, I'm pretty sure my nose is broken, and Scott's not giving in. I already put him down twice, but the stubborn bastard got back up each time.

I'm not worried. Just ready to be done now.

Round ten.

I take him to the ropes. Punch after punch after punch. The referee separates us. Bell goes. Scott is in his corner, glugging water. It's a sign he's tired. He's bleeding from the eye.

Round eleven.

I got him. He's mine now. I go in there, blazing. The Vaseline coating his cut isn't stopping the blood. It's in his eye. I see him lose focus, and that's when I strike. I hit him, uppercut. He goes down. And I know it's all over.

The referee is there, bending over him. Scott tries to get up. He can't.

The referee waves his hand, calling time on the fight.

And I've won.

My team floods the ring. Mike is hugging me. Then, Ares, Lo, and Missy are here, hugging me and telling me how proud they are of me.

But one voice is missing.

There's always one voice missing.

Hers.

My eyes do what they always do after every fight. They look for her. Like some part of my brain, even now, thinks she's going to be here.

Why would she be here?

You left her. She's not here because of you.

Then, the cameras are in front of me. Post-fight interview. Of course, Marcel is here for this. Always here for the cameras.

I thank my family. Thank Scott for the fight.

Marcel takes over, talking about himself—his favorite subject.

A commotion going on behind me catches my attention. I look over my shoulder. I can see people crowding around Scott. He's still on the floor.

What's going on?

I step away. Moving toward Scott.

Marcel stops me. "Where do you think you're going?" he grits out between clenched teeth.

"Scott is still down." I tip my head toward where he's on the floor.

"So?" is Marcel's response.

I hear a medic being called for. I go to move again,

Marcel tugs me back to the camera. "He's fine. Leave him."

I'm asked a question by the interviewer. I respond, half-distracted. Marcel starts talking about the fight.

I look back at Scott. The medic's there, bent over him, shining a flashlight in his eyes.

"Zeus," Marcel barks at me.

I ignore him this time. I pull away, quickly moving toward Scott again because I know this isn't right. He shouldn't have been down for this long. Something twists hard in my gut.

I push past the people crowding around Scott, almost reaching him, when I hear the words that will come to haunt me for the rest of my life.

"He stopped breathing. We need an ambulance. Now."

Chapter One

One Year Later

THAT FEELING . . . when the music is pumping, the bass pounding the floor beneath your feet, vibrating up your body . . . there's nothing like it.

Not for me anyway.

Dancing has always been my thing. I love it. And I'm damn good at it.

I trained in ballet and street dance. But I dropped street when I was a teenager, as ballet was always the dream. It was everything.

I was at Juilliard on a full scholarship, eyes set on the New York City Ballet. I was in my second year when everything changed.

Those two pink lines on the test changed everything. And my future changed into something else.

And, even now, up here on this podium, dancing my ass off like I do every Friday and Saturday night, I know I made the right decision.

And, no, before you ask, I'm not a stripper. I'm a go-go dancer at this upscale club in Manhattan.

Granted, this wasn't the stage I expected to be on when I was growing up. But life throws curveballs at you, and you have to go with them.

And my little curveball goes by the name Gigi, and I love her more than I imagined I ever could love anyone. She is the best decision I have ever made.

Okay, so she wasn't exactly planned.

I was on the pill, but I had been with her father for four years.

He was my childhood sweetheart. The absolute love of my life. I thought we'd grow old together.

Obviously, it didn't work out that way.

He dumped me. Over the phone.

Yes, he was in England at the time, and I was here, in New York, but hearing that the love of your life had cheated on you over the telephone isn't the best way to have things go down. And then to find out, a month later, that I was pregnant with his baby, only to have him tell me he didn't want anything to do with either of us—actually, he didn't even tell me himself; he got his manager, the great fucking Marcel Duran, to tell me and offer me money to go away, which I refused, of course—you could say, it has made me a little bitter about him.

But I have to be grateful for one thing—his donation of sperm—because it gave me Gigi, and she is the best thing that's ever happened to me.

The song currently playing, "Stay" by Zedd and Alessia Cara, comes to an end, and then Christina Aguilera's "Dirrty" blasts out from the speakers. The crowd goes nuts. And I'm thrown back fifteen years to nine-year-old me standing in front of the TV, watching the music video on MTV, trying to learn the dance moves to this song, and my aunt Elle joining in with me.

Aunt Elle doesn't have a rhythmic bone in her body. Great cop. Terrible dancer.

The memory makes me smile as I pump my body to the beat, pushing to excess, doing the dance routine my body remembers, even now from all those years ago.

I'm sweating. I've been dancing for a while now. Kim should be coming to take over soon. We always switch, doing twenty- to thirty-minute intervals.

I'm ready for a break, so I can recharge.

I push tendrils of hair off my face with my palm. My long brown hair is tied back in a high ponytail. I have naturally straight hair, but I have that overprocessed, shitty hair that goes frizzy without products and straighteners—hence the ponytail and stray hairs.

I feel a hand curl around my ankle, grabbing it. This isn't unusual for people, especially men, to get a little overly friendly. They think because I'm up here, dancing, that they have the right to touch me.

I look down and see a suit and a head of blond hair styled in that just-rolled-out-of-bed look that everyone knows he spent hours perfecting.

I meet his stare, and the telltale sign of too much alcohol is showing in the glaze of his eyes—well, that, and the beer bottle he's holding in his hand, which is forbidden on the dance floor.

I glance up and scan the area for security to alert them, but I can't see any of them. My eyes cut to the bar, but it's busy with customers, and I can't catch any of the bartenders to make eye contact.

For fuck's sake. Looks like I'm gonna have to handle this myself.

Keeping my expression friendly, I crouch down, putting me at eye-level with the handsy drunk. He's actually not bad-looking close up. Still doesn't give him the right to put his hand on me though.

I tap him on the hand. "No touching," I tell him kindly.

"Oh. Sorry." He removes his hand from my ankle.

See? Wasn't that easy? No security needed at all.

"No problem." I smile. Feeling generous toward the guy, I ask him, "Did you need something?"

He returns my smile—well, it's more of a grin—and then he says, "Yeah. You naked and in my bed, baby."

Ugh. And my good feeling toward him evaporates.

I resist the urge to roll my eyes.

If I had a dollar for every time I'd heard that line or one close to it, I'd be lying on a lounger right now in the back garden of my mansion in Beverly Hills, sunbathing by my Olympic-size swimming pool, with a Jason Momoa lookalike rubbing my feet in between serving me margaritas and servicing me (wink, wink) all day long.

"Yeah, not gonna happen, buddy." I laugh.

I go to stand up, but he snatches his hand out and grabs ahold of my wrist, keeping me there.

His grip is tight, and even though I'm surrounded by hundreds of people, I still feel that momentary spark of panic, but I fight it back down.

One good thing my ex did do, aside from giving me Gigi, was teach me how to defend myself. The plus side of dating a boxer for four years.

I stare him straight in the eye. "Let go of my arm."

"Aw, baby, don't be like that. I'm just being friendly." He flexes his fingers around my wrist.

"I think you need to go back to school and learn the meaning of the word. This is your last warning. My next one won't be so nice."

"I'd listen to her, if I were you."

Handsy Asshole lets go of my wrist and spins around to face the voice that just sent chills down my back. And not the good kind of chills.

My eyes cut up and over the head of Handsy Asshole, and for the first time in five years, I stare into the eyes of Zeus Kincaid.

The cheating bastard and heartless son of a bitch who walked away from me and his unborn child.

Aw, fuck to the hell no.

The shock of seeing him after all this time has his name rushing out of my lungs. "Zeus."

"Hi, Dove." His familiar deep voice saying the nickname he gave me all those years ago elicits a thousand memories. Good and bad.

I used to love it when he called me Dove.

Now, I hate it.

He called me it from the moment we met. Said I was like a dove. Beautiful and fragile. With my fight hidden inside me.

And, as time went on, Zeus said I was his peace in the chaos that was his life. I was his little dove.

And I believed him.

Until he decided he no longer needed his dove, and he stripped me of my wings and left me to die.

But I didn't die, and I got my wings back, too.

So, fuck you, Zeus.

"Hey . . . I know you." Handsy Asshole stares up at Zeus, pointing his finger at him.

Handsy isn't small by any means of the word. Probably about five eleven at a guess, but Zeus is bigger. Half a foot bigger to be exact. Six foot five and built of solid muscle.

And that's why he's the current heavyweight champion boxer of the world. That, and his God-given talent to hurt people. Most of the time, he doesn't even have to hit people to hurt them.

I'm living proof right here.

"Yeah, I know you. You're Zeus Kincaid, right? Holy shit! You are! I can't fucking believe it! Zeus fucking Kincaid. Dude, you're amazing! I won two Gs on your last fight. Hey, can I get a picture? My buddies aren't gonna believe this!"

Tearing my eyes from Zeus, I don't wait around to listen to his response. I use it as an opportunity to get the hell out of there.

Moving swiftly, I push up to stand, and I run down the steps off the podium. I quickly start making my way through the crowd, heading straight for the staff room.

My heart is pounding, my mind racing, and my feet can't move fast enough to get me out of there and away from Zeus.

I can't believe he's here.

I'm about ten steps away from the staff door, almost home free, when a hand curls around my biceps, bringing me to a stop.

I don't have to turn around to know who it is.

I tilt my face in Zeus's direction, tipping my head back to stare up into his face. I'm five nine—five eleven in my boots. Not short for a woman, but Zeus has always made me feel small.

I used to love that feeling.

Now, I hate it.

"What are you doing here?"

What am I doing here? That's it? That's all he has to say to me after five years of silence?

Not, *Did we have a boy or a girl?* Or, *How is my kid doing?*

God, I hate him.

I stare at him, wondering how I ever loved this man.

Zeus was always beautiful; there's never been any doubt about that. In the early days of his career, the press dubbed him The Pretty Boy of Boxing. I remember how much he hated that nickname. Nowadays, they call him The God.

I think he's The Devil.

But he's no longer the pretty-boy beautiful he was back then.

Now, he's ruggedly handsome. Even with the too-many-times broken nose and the scar that cuts through his eyebrow. I remember the fight in which he got that scar. It was over me. His trademark stubble on his cheeks, which I know is actually softer to the touch than it looks. And his dark hair, which he always wore shaved, is now styled—still short at the sides, but longer on top.

And his eyes . . . they were the first thing I noticed about him. If I had to give them a color, I'd say azure. The bluest of blue. Eyes with the depths of the ocean.

You stare into them, and they give away nothing but make you feel everything.

He might be physically stunning to look at, but inside of him is a totally different story.

He steps closer. His scent washes over me—familiar yet unfamiliar. He's changed his aftershave. He always used to wear Burberry Touch. It was my favorite aftershave. I used to buy it for him.

I guess he rid himself of everything that was me.

Including his child.

Something akin to a knife sticks in my heart.

"Dove, I asked you a question. What are you doing here?" His grip on my arm increases, his brows pulling together in frustration.

I see a hint of anger in his eyes. And it sparks me back to life.

He has the gall to demand an answer from me after what he's done.

Fuck. That.

I want to spit on him in disgust. But I don't. I keep my dignity—unlike the last time we spoke five years ago.

I fill my eyes with the contempt I feel for him, years' worth of hate and anger, and I grind out, "Don't call me that. My name is Cam. And what do you think I'm doing? I'm working, asshole."

I yank my arm from his hand and hurry to the staff room door. I punch in the code on the keypad, unlocking the door. I rush through it, letting it close behind me, to the sound of his voice calling my name.

Chapter Two

HANDS STILL SHAKING, I turn the key in the ignition, and my Toyota comes to life. Halsey's "Eyes Closed" bleeds out of the stereo. I drive out of the club's staff parking lot and start the hour journey home to Port Washington—to the home I share with Gigi and Aunt Elle. Technically, I still live at home, as it's Aunt Elle's house.

Aunt Elle moved to Port Washington from Coney Island when she got promoted to detective and was given a post at the precinct there. She could've commuted, but it seemed pointless, as I wasn't living at home anymore. I was at Juilliard and living in New York at the time.

But, when I found myself pregnant and alone, going to live with Aunt Elle was the only option. And, honestly, I was glad not to have to go back to Coney Island. The place held nothing but memories of Zeus and our relationship there. Also, I didn't want to risk running into any of his family there either.

So, Port Washington was my new start. And life has

been working out pretty well for me—well, up until a short time ago, that is.

I left work early. I had to get out of that place. So, I told my boss I was sick, and I needed to go home.

I couldn't risk going back out into the club and seeing Zeus again.

Seeing him after all these years . . . it's knocked me on my ass.

And the fact that he tried to talk to me . . . I just don't get it.

He made it perfectly clear that he wanted nothing to do with Gigi or me all those years ago, so why did he now come over to me and try to speak to me?

I'm just relieved that I won't have to see him again. I'm going to quit my job. He probably won't show his face at the club again, but I don't want to take the chance. My emotions can't take it.

I feel . . . I don't know how I feel. Angry. Hurt. Angry. Frustrated. Did I mention angry?

I'll just get another job at another club. It's not my main source of income anyway. I have a day job. I work admin at the police station.

I got the job at the club, so I could keep dancing. I put the money I earn into a savings account for Gigi for when she's older to pay for college or dance school, whichever she chooses. She's got the dance bug like her mama. And I know I'm biased, but she's good.

So, leaving there won't be the end of the world.

Seeing Zeus again would be.

The whole of my journey home is spent with me having internal arguments with myself.

Part of me thinks I should have said more to Zeus

tonight. That I should have said all the things I wanted to say to him five years ago but never got the chance. The smart side of me knows that I did the right thing, walking away and not looking back. But . . . I don't know.

I just know I want to get home and hug my daughter.

It hasn't been long since I passed the Welcome to Port Washington sign when blue lights flash in my rearview.

Flicking on my indicator, I slow my car down and pull over to the side of the road.

"If this is one of the guys screwing around, I'm gonna be pissed," I mutter to myself.

I could really do without this tonight.

I glance in my rearview, and in the dark, I see the officer getting out of his car and start walking toward mine.

I definitely wasn't speeding. I know that for a fact. But, if I have done something wrong, trust me, being the niece of Detective Reed won't get me out of a ticket. Not that I've tried and played that card.

Okay, well, maybe I have once or twice. But it's never worked.

I roll my window down and wait to see who it is. I know all the cops in this town. I've lived here for close to five years, but working at the station and having my aunt on the force means I've gotten to know all the cops.

"You're heading home early. Everything okay?"

I know that voice, and it brings a smile to my lips. Something I didn't think could happen tonight.

Rich Hastings is a guy I date. Well, maybe *date* is the wrong word. We hang out . . . in bed together.

Sometimes, in his shower. Or on his kitchen table. Anyway, you get the picture.

I'm not looking for a relationship, and neither is Rich.

After getting burned by Zeus, letting a guy into my life, and Gigi's, is not something I want to do.

Gigi thinks that Rich is just a guy Mommy works with. And he is. We also just happen to get naked together, too.

What I have with Rich works. We're on the same page. Sex, no strings. We have good chemistry. The sex is great. He's a nice guy. He makes me laugh. We have fun together.

I tip my face up to him. "Yeah, I'm fine. Just felt a bit tired, so I left early."

He leans down and puts his forearms on my car door, and I stare at his lovely face.

Rich is hot. Not Zeus hot. I don't think anyone could be. Zeus is on a different level to all other men. I hate that.

But Rich is attractive in that all-American boy kind of way. The exact opposite of Zeus. Blond hair. Green eyes. Six-two. Used to play college basketball. Athletic . . . hot. And he wears a uniform, so . . . you know, hot.

Rich's eyes go down and widen as he takes in my outfit, which is showing beneath my open coat.

I have to stifle a laugh. Men are so easy.

I didn't change out of my club clothes and into normal clothes like I usually do before heading home. I was in a rush to leave because of Zeus.

My club outfit consists of white PVC go-go boots, a hot-pink bandeau top, and matching hot pants. The outfits that the club has us wear don't leave much to the imagination.

"Nice outfit," he drawls. His dilated eyes land on my lips first and then on my eyes. "Why haven't I seen that one before?"

"Because you've never been to the club."

"Ah. My error. One I need to rectify immediately."

I laugh, but I don't really feel it, and I know exactly why.

Zeus.

Fucking Zeus.

"You sure you're okay?"

Rich cups my cheek in his hand, and I appreciate the warmth it brings.

I've been filled with so many different emotions since seeing Zeus—most of them bad—that I feel cold inside. I didn't realize just how cold until Rich put his hand on me.

Sometimes, it's the simplest of touches that can make you feel better. Well, maybe not better. I don't think I'll feel better for a while after running into Zeus tonight.

"I'm sure." I smile.

He brushes his thumb over my lips. "It's been a while since I've seen you," he says tenderly.

"I know. I've been busy with Gigi starting pre-K and work and life . . ."

"How's Gigi handling pre-K?"

"You know Gigi." I smile wide at the thought of my baby girl. "Nothing fazes her. She has the confidence of a seasoned performer."

"I wonder where she gets that from." He grins.

"I've no idea." I innocently flutter my lashes.

Rich chuckles and then leans in, gently kissing me on the lips.

It's sweet. It's nice.

He's not Zeus.

"I've missed you," he murmurs.

"You mean, you've missed being inside me."

He smiles against my mouth. "You could say that. When can I see you next?"

"How does Wednesday night sound? I'll ask Aunt Elle to watch Gigi."

"Wednesday sounds far away, but I'll take it." He leans back. "Guess I'm gonna be spending some more time with Rosie Palm and her five sisters." He grins, waving his palm at me, and I chuckle.

"You're a good-looking guy, Rich. I'm sure you're not wanting for women."

I don't know why I said that.

In the time we've been sleeping together, I've never asked Rich to be exclusive with me. It would be unfair when I can't give him a lot of my time. But I also never ask him about other women either.

Why would I say that now?

I know why.

Zeus.

The cheating, abandoning asshole has thrown me off-kilter.

Rich's brow goes up, and he leans his arms back on my window. "You saying you want me to sleep with other women?"

I think on that. I wouldn't say the thought of him with other women makes me explosive with jealousy, but it also doesn't make me feel particularly good either.

I shake my head, and he smiles.

"Do I need to be asking about other guys?"

That makes me laugh. "I barely have time for myself, so . . . no, you don't have to ask about other guys."

Except for the one I saw tonight.

Rich doesn't know who Gigi's father is. Only a few people do. And it's going to stay that way.

"I should take you out on a date."

That takes me aback. *What is it with men and them shocking the shit out of me tonight?*

"No, you shouldn't."

My smile is tight, and he nods in understanding.

He pushes back off my car, standing up straight. "Wear that on Wednesday." His eyes flick down to my outfit.

"Only if you wear that." I tip my head at his uniform.

"You got a deal." He steps back from my car. "See you Wednesday, Cam."

"See you." I restart my car. "Oh, and, Rich, have your handcuffs at the ready, too."

I give him a sexy smile.

"Yes, ma'am."

He winks and tips an imaginary hat at me.

I pull my car off the side of the road, a smile on my face. Then, the damn radio decides to play Rihanna's "Umbrella," and the smile slides off my face as I'm catapulted back nine years.

Chapter Three

Nine Years Ago

"EXCUSE ME."

I feel a tap on my shoulder and glance back to see a group of three girls standing behind me in line for the Ferris wheel.

They look my age. And they're cute and pretty in that dainty way I'll never be. I'm tall for my age, all long legs and arms. Perfect for ballet. Not so perfect for a teenager desperate to fit in.

Wanting to make new friends in this place I've just moved to, I smile and say, "Hi. Everything okay?"

One of them, who I'm guessing is the leader of the group, steps forward a little, closer to me. "Are you going on this alone?"

My cheeks heat. Because I am going on the ride alone. Not because I'm a total loser, but because we just moved to Coney Island from Baltimore. My aunt Elle is a police officer and she got offered a promotion, and that brought us here. I'd lived in Baltimore my whole life, so moving has taken a little getting used to. Okay, a lot getting used to. But Aunt Elle has done so much for me, raising me after my mom died when I was three, so when she told me about the promotion, I told her to go for it.

She's at work now, which is why I thought I'd come out and explore my new home. Instead of sitting at home, checking Facebook for what my friends back home were doing.

So, of course, I came to the famous fair. And I'm a sucker for the Ferris wheel. Hence, why I'm in line to ride.

"Yes. I'm new to town. I don't know anyone here," I tell her by way of explanation, partly hoping she'll invite me to join them on the ride.

She doesn't.

"Well, you do realize that those cars can take up to four people, and you're going to use one just on you. That's pretty selfish of you."

Wow. Okay.

"I'm not trying to be selfish. I just want to ride the Ferris wheel. Do you want . . . should I ride with you guys to fill the car up?"

She laughs. Then, she looks me up and down. "I don't think so. We don't hang out with losers. Right, girls?" She nudges her sidekicks, and they laugh along with her.

My face stings with humiliation. I should say, *Screw you then. You'll have to wait longer to go on the Ferris wheel because I'm going on it.* Or even flip them off.

But I do none of those things.

Instead, I walk out of the line to the sound of laughter and chants of, "Loser," my eyes stinging with tears.

What the hell is wrong with me? I should have given those bitches a piece of my mind.

Wrapping my arms around myself, I continue to walk. I suck in a breath, keeping my emotions from leaking out of my eyes.

I'm a Reed, and we don't take crap from anyone.

Or that's what Aunt Elle always says.

Honestly, I've never really had to put up with anything like that before. I had great friends back in Baltimore. And, now, I have no one.

I just know those girls will be at the high school I'm starting on Monday, too.

I stop outside a store across from an arcade, unsure of what to do with myself. The sounds of laughter, music, and the pinging machines dance in the air, making me feel even lonelier.

I'm gonna go home.

Well, back to the new house I now have to call home.

At least there's a tub of Cherry Garcia waiting for me in the freezer.

As I turn to leave, male laughter catches my attention, and I look to see a few guys standing around one of those boxing arcade games—you know, the kind where you hit the punching bag to record a high score.

One of them is having a turn. Something about him catches my attention even though his back is turned to me.

He's a big guy. Tall. Broad shoulders showcased in a blue denim jacket. My eyes go down. White T-shirt showing out of the bottom of his jacket. Black jeans on his legs. Nice ass. Fits his jeans well.

Fits his jeans well? Thank God I don't say this kind of crap out loud.

My eyes go back up. I can't see his hair, as he's wearing a ball cap.

I bet he's good-looking.

There's just something in the way he moves his body as he prepares to hit the punching bag that screams confident. Like he knows he's good-looking.

God, listen to me. I haven't even seen the guy's face, and I'm labeling him as hot.

He hits the bag hard. I could hear the slam of his fist against the leather of the bag, even all the way over here. The bag pounds up into the machine, and the board lights up with numbers running high.

Top score.

Wow.

His friends are laughing and punching him in the arm, like guys do, but he seems to just shrug them off.

Then, without warning, he turns his head and looks straight at me, catching me staring.

Shit.

I look away, turning to the store window. I use my long hair to curtain my face, trying to pretend I wasn't staring when he clearly knows I was.

I'm such a loser.

My face is reaching inferno levels of hotness at the embarrassment of getting caught staring and also because I was right. Holy Christ on a hottie cracker, that guy is gorgeous. Beautiful. The quick glimpse I saw of his face was more than enough to confirm to me that he is super high on the sex god meter. And definitely older than me. A lot older, I'd say. Around twenty-ish at a guess.

Yes, I know I'm a dork.

And I also look like a complete dick, standing here, staring into the window of a closed store. But I daren't turn around in case sex god is still there.

I can't hear him and his friends anymore, but that doesn't mean they're not there.

I look at the reflection in the store window to try to see if he and his friends are still there, but I can't.

Okay, so I'm just going to have to suck it up. Turn around and casually walk away like I wasn't just staring at the hottie.

One . . . two . . . three . . .

And they're gone.

I don't know whether to be relieved or disappointed that I'm probably never going to see the sex god again.

I stare at the boxing machine where he just was and have the sudden urge to try it before I head home. Not because sex god touched it. I'm not that much of a loser. I've just never tried one before, and I wonder if I'm any good.

I walk over to the arcade and stop at the boxing machine.

Fifty cents.

I dig into the pocket of my skinny jeans and pull out some coins.

I push them into the slot, and the machine lights up. The punching bag lowers.

I curl up my fist, ready.

Can't be that hard, right?

I pull my arm back and punch it.

Apparently, it is that hard.

Because I don't even move the bag back up to make a score. It just kind of wobbles a bit but stays put.

Well, that's embarrassing.

I glance around to see if anyone saw, but no one is paying me any attention.

Okay. Try again, Cam. You can do this.

I prepare myself a bit more this time.

I shake out my shoulders, loosening up. I spread my legs apart and plant my feet. Then, I swing my arm back and punch the bag.

Yay! I did it!

But . . . oh . . . is that the lowest score you can get?

Yep, that's me.

Right. I'm going again.

And, this time, I'm going to hit the crap out of this punching bag. It will not defeat me.

I get another fifty cents out of my pocket and drop the coins into the slot. The punching bag comes down.

"You're wasting your money."

"Wha—" I turn to the voice and—*holy shit.*

It's Sex God. He's standing right there. Looking at me.

Jesus. His eyes. Blue. Like the bluest of blue. The I-want-to-dive-into-them-and-never-again-come-up-for-air blue.

"Your stance is all wrong," he tells me. "You'll never get a good swing at the bag, standing like that." He nods at my legs.

I look down at them. *They look okay to me.*

"What's wrong with my legs?" I say.

He chuckles right as I hear those words echo back in my head, and I have to bite back a groan of embarrassment.

"Well, nothing's wrong with them." He lifts a shoulder.

"They're great legs. Best I've seen in fact. But the way you're standing isn't right. Your hips can't turn while you're standing like that, meaning there's no swing in your punch. No swing, no force."

Great legs.

Best he's seen.

Honestly, I didn't hear anything else after that.

"I'm sorry, what?"

He chuckles again. "You need to move your legs. Stand like this." He shows me with his own.

"Okay." I move my legs to mirror how he's standing.

"That's right," he tells me. "And, now, you need to tilt your hips back a little, like this."

I follow his instructions, tilting my hips.

"Then, put your hand into a fist, thumb on the outside. Pull your arm back, and let your hips pivot around. As you swing, put all your body weight into that punch."

I do as he said. I swing back and then put all my body weight behind my arm. Along with all my emotions from leaving Baltimore and my friends and from those mean girls from before.

I hit that bag with everything I have. I feel the moment my fist connects with the leather, and I get a good hit in.

The bag slams back up, and the numbers start to rise.

Medium hitter!

Yes!

"I did it!" I bounce on my toes, excited.

"You did." His lips lift at the corner into a half-smile. The sexiest smile I've ever seen.

And I'm a puddle at his feet.

I tuck my hair behind my ear. "Thanks," I say.

"No biggie." He shrugs.

"How do you know about boxing?" I ask him.

"I'm a boxer."

"Like, a real boxer?"

Kill me. Kill me now.

He smiles again. "Yeah, like, a real boxer. Well, I'm not pro. Amateur at the moment. I can't go pro until I get my boxing license, and I can't get that until I'm eighteen."

"You're not eighteen already?"

"Seventeen."

"Wow. You look much older."

He laughs. "I hear that a lot."

"So, you're a senior?"

"Junior. My birthday's in September."

"Ah. August baby here."

"Junior, too?"

"Nope. Sophomore. I'm fifteen," I add, like I need to highlight that fact to him.

Way to go, Cam. Turn him off with your age.

Not that he was turned on by me . . . but whatever.

He doesn't say anything for a long moment. I feel a stab of disappointment in my chest, which is crazy because I've only just met the guy.

"So . . . we're only one school year apart, but you're nearly two years older than me. Well, a year and eleven months older, which is weird if you think about it."

Jesus, Cam. Stop your rambling. Why don't you also tell him that your legal guardian is with the New York City Police Department and finish off any hopes you might have had with him.

"You look older," he says. "No offense."

"None taken. I hear that a lot, too. I think it's my

height. Hopefully, not my face. I don't want to have a prematurely aged face."

He laughs. But I don't feel like he's laughing at me, like he thinks I'm a total goof. More like he thinks I'm funny, in a good way.

And that does something funny to my stomach.

"You don't need to worry about your face," he tells me and smiles that half-smile again.

Something swoops up and flutters into my chest.

I feel giddy and light.

Goddamn, he's pretty.

"Where are your friends?" I ask, floating on a cloud of him.

"How did you know I was here with friends?"

Ah. Crap.

"I, um . . . well, I saw you before. You were on this game, and I was over there. But I wasn't stalking you or anything. I just saw you, is all."

I'm dying. Jesus. Kill me now.

He chuckles low and deep, and I feel it from the roots of the hair on my head to right down to the tips of my toes.

"I saw you, too," he tells me.

Wow.

Yeah . . . just wow.

"So, what are you doing now?" he asks me.

Going wherever you're going.

"Going home," I say.

"Why?"

"I have no clue." I'm fairly sure I can't even remember my own name right now.

"Then, you should stay."

"Why?" I hear myself asking.

That smile that turns me to Jell-O slides back onto his face.

"Good question. You want the truth?"

"Always."

He takes a step closer to me. His scent is spicy and something completely masculine, and it overwhelms me in the best possible way.

"Because I find you interesting. And usually nothing but boxing interests me. But you interest me."

"Why?" Apparently, that word is now two-thirds of my vocabulary.

"You're funny and pretty. Really pretty."

"And fifteen."

"And fifteen," he echoes.

"And my aunt is a cop."

"Good to know."

"Why?"

"Because it means you have someone looking out for you."

Oh.

"I'm not having sex with you, if that's what you're after."

Laughter bursts from him.

Filter, Cam. Filter, for God's sake.

"I was just thinking of a walk. Maybe a ride on the Ferris wheel. But good to know where your head's at." He wipes the laughter from his eyes.

"Sorry," I say.

"Don't be. You're right to be careful. You don't know me." He pauses and lifts his cap from his head. His hair is dark brown. He runs his hand over his sheared hair.

Then, he puts his cap back on and fixes those bright blue eyes of his on mine. "But I want you to know me. And I really want to know you."

I bite my lip and then tuck my hair behind my ear. "Okay," I say.

He smiles. A full smile this time, showing his teeth. They're white but not perfect. His front teeth have a slight overlap to them. But it suits him. Makes him even more handsome, if that's possible.

"I'm Zeus," he tells me.

"Like the god?"

He chuckles, and I realize how that sounded.

"Not that I think you're a god, of course," I add with a roll of my eyes to try to come off as nonchalant. It totally doesn't work.

"Of course not." He smiles. "But, yeah, like the god."

"Cameron. But everyone calls me Cam."

"Who's everyone?"

"My aunt."

"The cop."

"And my friends back home in Baltimore. I just moved here a few days ago."

He nods, like he already knows this. "Have you been on the Ferris wheel yet?" he asks.

I shake my head, not wanting to say that I wanted to but didn't because of a couple of mean girls.

"Well, you can't come to the fair and not go on the Ferris wheel. It's like the law of Coney Island."

"Really?" I lift a skeptical brow.

"No." He grins boyishly, and I laugh. "But you do need to go on the Ferris wheel. Come on." He holds his hand out to me.

"Um . . ." I hesitate, and he sees it.

"Do you not like Ferris wheels?"

"No. I mean, yeah, I do. I just . . . well, without sounding like a kindergartener, I was in line to ride it just before, and . . . some girls were mean to me. And, after that, I didn't so much feel like going on it anymore."

"How were they mean?"

"I can't believe I'm telling you this." I self-deprecatingly roll my eyes, exhaling a breath.

But he doesn't say anything. Just waits.

So, I say, "They called me a loser because I was going to go on the ride alone."

"And do you care what they think?"

"Yes. I mean, no. Kind of. It's stupid. I'm stupid."

"No, you're not. Look, people like that are just shitty because they're insecure themselves, and they need to try to bring everyone else down to make them feel better about themselves."

"Are you speaking from experience?"

"No. I'm just smart." He grins, and I smile. "Look, don't let some mean girls put you off from doing something you want to do."

I stare up at him. Not many guys make me feel small and girlish, but he does.

"You're right," I tell him.

"I know. I usually am." Another half-smile. "And, anyway, you won't be alone this time. I'll be with you."

My eyes narrow a touch. "You're not going to try to murder me on the Ferris wheel, are you?"

Another burst of laughter from him.

"It wasn't on my agenda for tonight, no." His eyes are shining and flickering like blue flames.

"And you're not gonna try to cop a feel?"

"Nope. I'll be the perfect gentleman." He lifts his hands up, palms facing me.

"Okay then, let's do it." I nod. "Ride the Ferris wheel, that is."

"You got it, Dove."

"Dove?" I blink up at him.

"Yeah. Doves represent peace because they look beautiful and appear gentle and fragile. But they're actually feisty as hell. They have more fight in them than people realize. Just like you."

Beautiful. He said doves are beautiful. Does that mean he thinks I'm beautiful?

Calm your jets there, Cam. Just because he said that does not mean he thinks you're beautiful.

I give him a look of amusement. "Wow. You got all that from a five-minute conversation."

"Nope." He shakes his head, a smile in his eyes. "I got all *that* from the way you hit the bag."

He sets off walking. I fall into step beside him.

"So, how come you know so much about doves?"

He slides me a look. "I don't. I just saw it on a nature show once."

I let out a laugh, and he grins.

We walk to the Ferris wheel in comfortable silence, and I muse to myself at how things are so different from when I was walking away from this ride not so long ago.

We join the line, which is much shorter than before. And there are no mean girls in sight.

Zeus insists on paying for me, which is really sweet.

We walk up to the car. The fairground attendant holds the door open for us.

Zeus gets in first. Then, he holds his hand out to me to help me in.

I hesitate for a second, and then I slip my hand into his. I know this is going to sound cheesy and clichéd, but I swear, the moment my skin touches his, it's like everything changes.

The world suddenly looks a lot brighter. The noises a little louder.

Like I was experiencing life in 2-D, and I've just upgraded to 3-D.

I sit next to Zeus, letting go of his hand, and the attendant shuts the door, securing us in.

We move up for the next car to be filled. Going up and around as each car fills for the actual ride. Dusk quickly turns to dark.

Then, we're moving.

"So, you live with your aunt?" Zeus's voice moves through the dark, making the hair rise on my arms in the best possible way.

"Yeah. My mom died when I was three, and my dad wasn't around, so my aunt Elle took me in. She's great."

"She sounds it. Sorry about your mom."

I shrug. "I don't remember her, so I don't remember losing her. But I don't remember having her either, which is what sucks most."

"Yeah . . ." His voice sounds pensive. "But maybe it's not such a bad thing—not having to feel the pain of losing her, you know."

"Yeah, I know what you mean. Anyway, sorry to bring the mood down." I turn my face to him.

"You haven't." He gives me a gentle smile.

"What about you?" I ask.

"What about me?"

"Parents? Brothers and sisters?"

He stares ahead. "Dad. My mom died last year."

Ah.

His solemn observation makes a lot more sense now.

"Shit. Sorry." I wince.

"Don't be." He shrugs. "She had been sick for a long time. Cancer."

"Fuck cancer, right?" It's all I can think of to say, but it must be the right thing because he looks back at me, a small smile touching his lips.

"Yeah, fuck cancer," he agrees.

"What about brothers and sisters?"

"Two brothers. One sister."

"Wow. That must be awesome."

"That's not the word I'd use." He chuckles.

"I would love to have siblings."

"You can have mine if you want."

I laugh. "If only. Tell me about them."

"Ares is two years younger than I am."

"Like me."

"Yeah. Like you," he echoes. "And the twins, Apollo and Artemis, are twelve."

"You all have Greek gods' names," I say and then cringe. "And I'm clearly on fire tonight with my blatant observations."

He laughs, and I realize that I really like the sound. A lot. And I want to keep on hearing it even if at my own expense.

"So, any reason for the choice of names?" I ask him. "I know some parents call their children names like River and Grass because they're hippies."

"My parents met in a Greek mythology lecture when they were at college. My dad's lame pick-up line was that if he and my mom had a kid together, they should call him Zeus 'cause with my mom's beauty and brains and my dad's size, their kid would be godlike. Clearly, she fell for it because here I am." He spreads his arms.

"And are you?"

"What?" He turns his face to me.

"Godlike?" *Because, from where I'm sitting, you sure as hell look like one.*

Zeus's eyes hold mine for a long time. "No," he says softly. "I bleed just like everyone else, Dove."

The ride comes to a stop, leaving us stationary at the top.

"Ride must be over," Zeus muses, looking over the edge. "They're letting people off."

I feel a spike of sadness that it's almost to the end. I could stay on here with him for ever.

Something wet hits my nose. Then, my forehead.

"Is it raining?" I say right as the heavens open. I mean, they open wide. It's pouring down.

"I'd say so." Zeus laughs.

"Jesus! I'm getting soaked!"

The shelter over the top of the car is doing nothing to shield us. I can hear the other people on the wheel squawking out their dismay over the sound of the music playing.

"Come on. Move, Mr. Ferris Wheel," I chant, now wishing for the ride to hurry up so that I can get off it and under some shelter.

Zeus pulls off his jacket. "Here, put this over your head," he offers.

"You'll get soaked."

"I'm fine. It's just a bit of rain."

"Share it?"

"Okay."

He holds the jacket over our heads, and I have to move in a little closer to get us both under the shelter.

I look up, and his face is so close to mine. I can see the droplets of water on his face. Feel the heat of his breath on my cheek.

I somehow register the song that's currently pumping out of the speakers on the ground below.

"Do you think it's a little ironic that 'Umbrella' is playing while it's raining like the Great Flood is about to start?"

He purses his lips in the most adorable way. "That, or fate."

"Fate?"

"Mmhmm."

"How so?"

He's staring at my lips, and it's making my heart beat faster. My pulse is racing off, sending adrenaline shooting through my veins.

His gaze lifts to mine. "I have no clue."

He smiles, eyes dancing with humor, and I laugh.

God, he's gorgeous. And I can't stop staring at him.

My breaths are coming in shallow pants, and I notice his are, too.

I inhale, and my lungs fill with him. That heady, spicy smell of his mixed in with the cool scent of rain does crazy things to me. Hormones are setting off inside me like rockets.

Water trickles down his cheek, catching on his upper lip.

And I really want to catch those raindrops with my lips.

So, I do.

I don't know what comes over me, but without a second thought, I lean in and press my lips to his.

Shit. I'm kissing him!

And . . . he's not kissing me back.

I make a strangled sound in my throat as I pull back at the realization of what I've just done.

I kissed him, and he didn't kiss me back.

Can I please die now?

God, I'm so freaking dumb. Of course he's not interested in me in that way. He's older and gorgeous. He could have anyone.

"Oh God," I groan, covering my face with my hands. "I'm so sorry, Zeus. After my big don't-try-to-cop-a-feel lecture, I attack you with my lips. I really don't know why I did that." *Well, I do. He's hot, and I'm stupid.* "Can we just pretend that never happened?"

"No."

My heart pauses. "No?" I lower my hands from my face.

The shield of his jacket is now gone, and he's staring at me with this intensity in his eyes that makes my toes curl up in my sneakers.

"No." He slides a hand around my cheek, cupping my face. "Even if I did want to pretend it never happened, which I don't, I wouldn't be able to. Because it's scorched in my memory."

"Scorched in your memory in a good way?"

"The best way."

He smiles, and I feel like I'm falling or floating or something.

Rain trickles onto my lips. He catches it with his thumb, making me shiver.

His eyes focus there, and my insides are swirling like a whirlpool.

"Are you going to kiss me?" I whisper.

"I want to . . ."

"I hear a *but.*"

His eyes lift to mine. "You're fifteen. And I'm seventeen."

All my good feelings come to a halt. "And?"

Silence stretches between us.

He hasn't stopped looking at me, and I don't know what this means or what I'm feeling. All I know is that I want to be with him. This guy I've known for only a short period of time. But he's making me feel things I've never felt before, and I want to keep feeling them.

"And"—his lip lifts at the corner, giving me that gorgeous smile of his—"we'll take it slow, Dove."

Chapter Four

"WHOA! SLOW DOWN, GIGI."

My little ballerina comes flying past me in the kitchen, doing a running leap, and I catch hold of her and scoop her up into my arms. She wraps her tiny legs around my waist.

"Mommy." She frowns at me, disapproving, that cute little dimple appearing between her beautiful brows. "I was *pwacticing* my leaps."

"I know what you were doing, Gigi girl, and it's good to practice." I tweak her nose with my thumb and finger. "But the kitchen is not the place to do it. And you're going to be at ballet class in thirty minutes, so you'll be doing lots of practice then."

"We need a dance studio here, so I can *pwactice* all the time."

I smile at her. "Now, wouldn't that be something?"

"Can we have one?"

Her face lights up, and I chuckle.

"No, Gigi girl. Maybe if we lived in a mansion, but not here, in Granny Elle's house."

She twists in my arms, turning her face to Aunt Elle, who's standing at the counter, making coffee. "Granny Elle, can I have a dance studio here, *pwease*?"

Aunt Elle comes over and takes her from my arms. Gigi wraps herself around her like a blanket.

"*Pwease*, Granny Elle. I *weally, weally* want one." She plants her hands on Aunt Elle's cheeks and gives her doe eyes.

She has Zeus's eyes. Big and blue and hard to say no to.

"Of course you can." Aunt Elle folds like a pack of cards.

"Yay!" Gigi squeals, and I groan. "Granny Elle, you da best!" She smacks a kiss to her cheek. Then, she wriggles out of Aunt Elle's arms and runs out of the kitchen.

"Stop running! And don't mess your hair up or get your clothes dirty! And get your ballet shoes from your room. We're leaving soon!" I call after her.

"You know that girl isn't listening to a word you say, right?" Aunt Elle chuckles.

"Yep. Because someone just promised her a dance studio in the house." I give a pointed look, and Aunt Elle laughs again.

"She's impossible to say no to. Especially when she's dressed up, all cute, in her ballet clothes. She reminds me of you at that age. Guess I'll just have to convert the dining room into a dance studio for her."

I bark out a laugh. "Yeah, and we'll eat in the living room, balancing our dinners on our knees. Why do you have such a problem saying no to her? You never had any problem saying no to me when I was growing up."

Aunt Elle pours me a coffee and hands me the mug. I take it from her.

"Because you're my kid, Cam. It's easier to say no to your own kid. Grandkids, impossible."

My heart always swells to combustion when she says things like that. And feeling emotional after last night's events, I put my coffee down on the counter and wrap my arms around her.

"I love you," I tell her.

She presses a kiss to my temple. "Love you, too, girl."

As I move back, she takes my face in her hands and stares into my eyes. "Everything okay with you?"

I bite my lip and shake my head. "I saw Zeus last night," I say quietly. "He was at the club."

A multitude of emotions flashes through her eyes. Anger being the main one. "That's why you were home early last night."

"Did I wake you when I came in?"

"I was in bed, reading. I never sleep until you're home. You should know that by now."

I touch my hand to hers. Then, I step back from her, pick up my coffee, and take a sip.

"Did he speak to you?"

I nod.

"What did he say?"

"He asked what I was doing there."

She frowns. "At the club?"

"Yes."

"And what did you say?"

"I said that I was working."

"Did he ask about . . ." Aunt Elle nods in the direction of the door where Gigi just disappeared through a minute ago.

I let out a heavy sigh and put my cup down. "No."

Her eyes blaze, nostrils flaring. "That mother . . . effing . . . craptastic . . . A-hole!" Aunt Elle whispers out her fire.

We're a curse-free zone here. Gigi has the ears of a bat and the voice box of a parrot. She hears and repeats everything. And I mean, everything.

"I'm not surprised, Aunt Elle. You shouldn't be either. He made his feelings perfectly clear five years ago."

"I know, but still . . ." She grits her teeth. Jaw working angrily.

"It doesn't matter. *He* doesn't matter."

"No, he doesn't. You and Gigi have done just fine without him," Aunt Elle adds.

"Yeah," I agree. *But Gigi shouldn't have had to*, I silently add.

Aunt Elle puts some bread in the toaster.

"Can you put a slice in for me? I'm just gonna go grab Gigi's ballet shoes and get her ready to leave."

"Sure thing."

I stop at the kitchen door. "You want to go out for dinner tonight?" I ask her. "You, me, and Gigi. Girls' night?"

"You're not working at the club?"

"No. I think I'm gonna quit. Just in case . . . you know."

Her face softens. "I know. And I'd love to go out for dinner with my girls. Where are you thinking?"

"DiMaggio's?" I suggest.

"Italian's always good." She smiles.

"Oh, and I need to ask for a favor. Would you mind watching Gigi for a few hours on Wednesday night?"

"Sure. No problem. You seeing Rich?"

"Mmhmm." My cheeks redden a little.

Aunt Elle knows about my arrangement with Rich. She doesn't pass judgment. Probably because she saw what I went through with Zeus. That, and she's never had a serious relationship in her life.

"Married to the job," she always tells me.

"I won't go out until she's in bed."

"Cam, you should go out. And not just to Rich's for a booty call."

"Please never say that again," I groan, slapping a hand to my face.

She laughs. "Go out and enjoy yourself. Get Rich to take you out for dinner or drinks."

Okay, so I take it back. She *never* used to interfere. I'm wondering if me seeing Zeus last night has set this off.

"We don't do that," I tell her. "And I go out enough."

She turns, facing me, and rests her hip against the counter. "You should do that. Rich likes you. A lot. I can tell. He's always asking me about you. He's a good guy, Cam. He'd take care of you."

"You mean, he's not Zeus."

"No, he isn't. You need to start living your life, Cam."

"I am living it." I defensively fold my arms.

"Your life centers around Gigi. And that's great. It should. You're an amazing mother. But you don't do anything for yourself. You don't go out. You don't date. And I know it's because of him and what he did."

"You haven't committed to a man," I cut her off. "You never had a man in your life while I was growing up. And you still don't now."

She sighs and runs a hand through her long, dark

hair. "But that's not because of what someone did to me. The moment I became a cop, I married my job. And, when you came to me . . . you needed me. The life you had with your mom . . . God, I loved my sister, Cam. And I don't want to speak ill of your mom, but she didn't do right by you. She was an addict. She moved you around all the time. Let different men in and out of her life. I tried to help her, get her clean, but she wouldn't listen. She fought me at every turn. She was too far gone for me to help her. But you weren't. And, if I'm being honest here, I was going to go after custody of you anyway if she hadn't died."

I suck in a breath. "You've never told me that."

She lifts a shoulder. "I loved you. And I wanted you safe. You needed security and stability, Cam. I'm married to the badge. I had room for only one person in my life back then, and it was you."

I can feel myself getting weepy. I'm not usually this emotional, but seeing Zeus last night has really knocked me off course.

Aunt Elle walks over, standing before me, and takes hold of my long hair, smoothing it over my shoulders. "I just want you to have something for yourself," she says.

"I dance," I say softly.

"At the club, which is work. I just want you to go out this once, let your hair down, and have fun."

"Okay," I concede. "I'll go out for drinks with Rich. Happy?"

She smiles winningly. "Yep."

I roll my eyes right as the doorbell rings. "I'll get it," I tell her.

After I walk out of her embrace, I stop and look back

at her. "I know I don't call you Mom, but I think of you as my mother. You know that, right?"

Her expression goes tender. "I know."

The doorbell rings again.

"Christ. Impatient much? Coming!" I yell.

I walk out of the kitchen, heading for the front door, and I pass the stairs. "Gigi, you got those ballet shoes yet? We're leaving in a few minutes."

"I'm getting them now!" Her voice sounds high-pitched and squeaky, and it only gets that way when she's doing something she shouldn't be.

I pause at the foot of the stairs. "Gigi?"

The bell rings again.

I look over my shoulder at the door and yell, "I'm coming!" Then, my eyes go back to the stairs. "Giselle Grace Reed, get your cute little butt down here right now."

She appears at the top of the stairs, stepping out from behind the wall.

"Oh, for the love of all that is holy. Gigi!"

I'm guessing what was my new red lipstick is now smeared all over her face. She looks like a clown.

"What were you thinking?"

She shrugs. "I'm sorry, Mommy. But it was just there, and it was so *pwetty*. I'm *weally* sorry."

I pinch the bridge of my nose. "Go in the bathroom. I'm gonna answer the door, and then I'll be there to help you wash it off."

She hightails it off to the bathroom. I mutter a few choice words under my breath and head for the front door.

I bend down and pick up the mail. Then, I unlock

the door and swing it open, and my heart stops. "Jesus!" The mail drops from my hand, scattering to the floor.

His lip lifts at the corner, giving me his trademark half-smile. "Well, I still go by Zeus, but you can call me Jesus if you like."

Chapter Five

"How about I call you nothing, and you get the hell off my porch? How does that sound?"

His hands lift in surrender. "I just want to talk, Cam."

"We have nothing to talk about. Except maybe how the hell you know where I live."

"Mommy!"

Gigi.

Fuck.

"I'll be there in a minute, baby," I call back. I can hear the tremor in my voice. I just hope he can't.

I quickly step outside, onto the porch, and pull the door closed behind me.

I look back to Zeus. He's looking beyond me, at the door. But I recognize the expression in his eyes.

Pain.

And that just makes me angrier.

"You need to leave, Zeus. Now."

His eyes flash down to mine. "Cam—"

But he's cut off when the door flies open behind me.

"Mommy, I got it off! All by myself! See? I used wet wipes and the *wipstick* came *wight* off."

My eyes swing down to Gigi. She's still got lipstick marks on her face. But I can't focus on that. Because her father is standing right there, in front of her, and she has no clue who he is.

Anger twists my gut.

I feel helpless and hurt and fucking livid.

I don't know what to do. All I do know is that I want to get Gigi away from him, so he can't hurt her like he hurt me.

But, before I even get the chance to get her back inside, she spots him.

"Who are you?" She steps forward, squeezing beside me, and tips her head back. Her eyes—*his* eyes—stare up at him in question.

My stomach drops out. "He's no one," I say quickly before he can speak. "Just the new mailman. You go back inside, Gigi. I'll be in there in a sec."

"We have a new mailman? Aw, but I *wiked* our old one. He told funny jokes. Do you tell funny jokes, New Mailman?"

I look up to Zeus, who is staring down at Gigi. His brow is creased. The way it always got when he was puzzled. When he couldn't quite figure something out.

He shakes his head without taking his eyes from her. "I don't know any jokes, kid. Sorry."

Kid. He called her kid. Like he doesn't even know her.

But he doesn't.

I think I'm going to throw up.

"Gigi girl, can you go inside, please?" I say.

She ignores me and carries on. "S'okay," she says to

him with a shrug. "I'll teach you some. I know lots. So, what's your name, Mr. Mailman? Our old one was called Burt. My name's Giselle Grace Reed. Everyone calls me Gigi. I have my granny Elle's name. She's called Giselle, too, like me, but everyone calls her Elle. And I have my other granny's name, too—Grace—but I've never met her. She's in heaven, Mommy says."

Zeus's eyes snap up to mine. Something in his expression twists.

"Gigi, please go inside, baby." This time, I usher her into the house with my hands. "Get Granny Elle to help you find your ballet shoes."

"Aw, but, Mommy, I was talking to our new mailman."

"Gigi," I say, using my mommy voice, "do as I asked."

She sighs in that dramatic way she does. "Fine. Bye, Mr. Mailman." She waves at him and then disappears back into the house.

I shut the door behind me and turn back to Zeus. His expression is tight. His eyes on the door. The spot where Gigi just was. Like he's still watching her.

I step up to him, blocking his view, and hiss out, "You need to leave right the hell now. You have no goddamn right, turning up here like this."

His eyes flash to mine. They look raw and angry and confused.

But I'm not confused. I know what I want, and it's him, gone.

"Grace." His voice sounds like gravel. He swallows. "She said her grandmother's name is Grace . . . *my* mother's name. And her eyes, Cam . . . so fucking blue . . . exactly like mine."

"Of course they're like yours!" I explode. "I can't believe you think you can turn up here after all these years and just—"

"Stop!" His loud voice booms through the air, cutting me dead. "You said, of course her eyes are like mine." His eyes are flickering between confusion and panic, and it's making me jittery. "Are you telling me . . . are you saying . . . she's my kid?"

My anger level leaps from fifty to a hundred in naught-point-one-second. "Are you fucking kidding me right now?" I yell.

"Do I look like I'm joking?" he bellows.

The door opens behind me.

"Enough." Aunt Elle's voice comes from behind me. "If I can hear you, then Gigi can hear you. You need to leave, Zeus."

"Not until I get answers."

"You want me to sling your ass in jail? 'Cause, honestly, it'd be a pleasure after everything you put Cam through."

"Put me in jail?" He laughs a sound of disbelief. "Are you shitting me right now? Cam has been keeping my kid from me, and you're giving me shit? What a fucking joke."

"I did what?" I screech. "It was you who wanted nothing to do with her!"

Zeus turns his flaming eyes on me. "How could I say that when I didn't even know she existed?"

"Stop it. Now. The both of you. Gigi doesn't need to hear this." Aunt Elle turns to me. "Cam, I'll take Gigi to ballet. You and Zeus talk. Because it's clear you need to." She yanks open the door and calls inside, "Gigi girl, I'm taking you to ballet. Grab your bag, and let's go."

"Coming!" Gigi comes happily skipping through a few seconds later, thankfully unaware of what's been happening out here.

Gigi looks up at me. Her happy expression dims at whatever she sees on my face. "You 'kay, Mommy?"

I clear my expression and paste on a smile. "Yeah, I'm fine, baby girl. I just need to speak to the new mailman, is all, so Granny Elle's going to take you to class."

"He forget the mail?" Gigi frowns.

I glance up at Zeus, who's not looking at me. His eyes are fixed on Gigi. My stomach balls into knots.

"Yeah, he forgot the mail. But don't you worry. You go have fun at ballet." I lean down and cup her chin in my hand. I kiss the tip of her nose. "I love you."

"I *wove* you, Mommy."

"Come on, let's get in the car," Aunt Elle says, grabbing her keys from the key hook by the door.

"Bye, Mommy. Bye, Mr. Mailman." She waves and starts skipping toward Aunt Elle's car parked on our driveway.

"You going to be okay?" Aunt Elle checks before leaving.

"I'll be fine." I nod.

"I've got my cell with me, if you need me." She turns her eyes on Zeus. "I'll be back in an hour. If I find out you've upset her again or hurt her in any way, then I'm coming after you with my shotgun. You hear me, Kincaid?"

Zeus works his jaw. "I hear ya."

"Good."

Aunt Elle gives me a quick hug, and then she goes over to her car and gets in.

I watch her and Gigi drive away, not wanting to look at Zeus.

When I do, his burning eyes are on me.

"She's mine."

"Of course she yours! Did you not get the memo the first two times?"

"What the fuck are you talking about?"

I realize we're both yelling again, and I don't want the neighbors knowing my business.

"I'm not doing this out here with you. Come inside."

I open the door, standing aside while he steps in. I shut the door behind him and lean against it.

He's an imposing figure in our little hallway. Zeus was always big. But, looking at him now, in the light of day, he looks even bigger than he did five years ago.

"She's mine? I have a daughter. How could you? Jesus, Cam."

"How could I, what?"

"Jesus, I know I hurt you . . . but keeping my kid from me? How could you do that?"

"What?" I straighten up, my eyes bugging out of my head. "I think you're a little confused here. I did not keep Gigi from you. You said you wanted nothing to do with either of us!"

"Was I fucking asleep when that conversation happened?" he yells, taking a step toward me.

Any other person might be intimidated by this move from him. But not me. I know Zeus. I know he'd never physically hurt me. Still, it doesn't stop me from shuddering inside.

"You need to back the fuck up." I jab my finger in his chest. "And how the hell should I know what you were doing when I couldn't get in contact with you? I tried to call your cell, and you'd either blocked my number or changed it. I even tried e-mailing you, asking you to call me, but they all went undelivered. So, I called Marcel. I knew he would be able to get me in touch with you. He took my call. Said you didn't want to talk to me. I told him that it was important. But he wasn't listening, so I told him that I was pregnant. Then, he started listening. He said he'd have you call me. And the rest you know."

"No, I don't. I don't know a fucking thing. What is the rest, Cam?"

"Are you being serious right now?"

"As serious as a heart attack."

"Oh God. Jesus. You didn't know . . . about Gigi?"

"No. But Marcel knew, right?"

I nod my head, watching as his face darkens like a thundercloud. "He called me back. Said that he'd talked to you. Told me he was sorry, but you'd said that you wanted nothing to do with the baby—our baby. That you'd support it financially, but that was it."

His eyes close, as if the pain is too hard to control.

"Marcel never told you, did he?" I say softly.

"No."

"Jesus. All this time . . . you didn't know. I . . ." Words are failing me. This entire time, I thought he'd walked away from Gigi, and he'd had no clue that she existed.

Zeus backs up and sits down on the stairs, like standing is just too hard for him right now. He covers his face with his hands as he takes deep breathes in and out. "I can't believe Marcel did this. I'm gonna fucking kill him. With my bare hands. Jesus! Fuck!"

I don't say anything. I'm trying to take this all in myself.

I hated him for leaving her, and he never even knew she existed.

My eyes close on the reality of the situation. I take a few deep breaths, trying to steady myself.

When I open my eyes, Zeus is staring up at me. Emotions are glistening in his eyes.

"She's really mine," he says more to himself than me. "Jesus, Cam, I have a daughter."

"Yes."

"Fuck." His hands cover his face again, and he blows out a harsh breath.

"Can I get you anything? Coffee? Brandy? I hear it's good for shock."

He draws his hands from his face. "Coffee's fine."

Hands shaking, I tell Zeus to take a seat in the living room while I go make us some coffee.

There's still some in the pot from before. I grab two cups and pour the drinks, leaving his black, just like he likes it. I put some creamer in mine and then carry the drinks through.

When I come into the living room with our coffees, I find Zeus standing at the fireplace, the framed picture I have of Gigi up there in his hands.

"Hey, your coffee," I say, putting the cups down on the coffee table between us.

He turns to me, the picture still in his hand. "I can't believe she's mine."

My spine stiffens. "She is. We can do a paternity test if you want the proof."

He fixes me with a stare. "That's not what I meant, Cam."

I blow out a breath. "Sorry."

I sit down on the sofa. Zeus walks over and sits down next to me, still holding the picture.

"She's beautiful," he says. "She looks just like you."

It's hard to have him here, so close, hearing him say that, after all these years. Especially with the hurt and resentment I've felt for him for so long, and in many ways, I still do feel it.

He didn't know about Gigi. I know that now.

But he did sleep with someone else while he was still mine.

"I don't know. I think she looks like Aunt Elle."

"You look like Elle," he says, making his point.

"Yeah, well, she has your eyes," I tell him. "And your smart mouth."

That makes him smile. "Does she know . . . about me? That she has a dad? I mean, everyone knows they have a dad, but does she know who her dad is?"

I shake my head.

"Can I . . . I want to know her. Spend time with her. Get to know my daughter, Cam."

My heart stops. I know I should have expected this. But I wasn't prepared for it.

"I . . . I don't know, Zeus. She's in a good place. She's happy. I don't want to upset her life."

"Neither do I. But please, Cam, I want to know my

daughter. I know I've messed up in the past . . . but I have to know her. She's my flesh and blood."

The desperation in his voice tightens my throat.

"I don't know . . ." I'm scared that he'll hurt her. That he'll walk away from her without a backward glance.

"I'll do anything, Cam. Take this as slow as we need to. But please don't keep me away from my daughter."

I close my eyes and take a deep breath.

"Please, Dove."

I open my eyes and look at him. "Okay."

He visibly exhales with relief. "Thank you."

"But you can't screw this up, Zeus."

"I won't."

"And we take this slow. Gigi doesn't know you. You're a stranger to her."

He winces.

"Christ, I'm sorry. I didn't mean that to sound so harsh."

"Don't be sorry. It's not your fault. None of this is."

"Maybe it is. I should have pushed harder to get Marcel to let me talk to you. Or contacted your family . . ."

"It's not your fault," he reinforces. "I cut you off. Made it so you had no way of contacting me."

It's my turn to wince with pain. But I keep it hidden inside of me.

"I thought it would be for the best . . ." His voice peters out.

"It's the past. Can't change it."

"No," he says. Then, he takes a breath and looks at me. "So, how do we do this? Me getting to know my daughter."

It's weird to hear him calling her that. But she is his daughter, and he deserves to know her.

"Well, I guess we'll introduce you as a friend to start with, so as not to upset and confuse her, and you can spend time getting to know one another. Then, when the time is right . . . we'll tell her who you really are."

"Her dad," he says.

"Yeah. Her dad."

Chapter Six

"WILL YOU TELL ME about Gigi?" Zeus asks me.

"Of course. What do you want to know?"

He stands the picture on the coffee table and angles his body toward mine. "Everything." He gives me a weak smile.

"Okay, so she's smart as a whip. Loves to dance—ballet mostly. But she enjoys tap and street, too. She loves *My Little Pony.* All things Disney. Her favorite Disney princess is Rapunzel, and she wants to marry Flynn Rider when she's older."

Zeus chuckles. "I have no idea who that is."

"Don't worry." I smirk. "You will soon."

"When's her birthday?"

"April 6."

"What was she like as a baby?"

"She was really good. Super cute, of course."

"Of course." He smiles.

"You want to see pictures?"

His eyes brighten. "Sure, if that's okay."

"Of course it is. Just wait a minute, and I'll grab them."

I rise to my feet and move past Zeus. He catches hold of my hand, and I freeze. His big hand is engulfing mine. I used to love the feel of his fingers around mine. Now, I just feel confused and hurt. And a million other things I shouldn't be feeling.

"Cam," he says softly.

I stare down at him. His eyes are searching and soulful as they look into mine. And it hurts like a bitch.

"I'm sorry," he says gently, carefully. "For everything."

I shrug like it doesn't matter. But it does. Because his apology only opens up old wounds, and it doesn't change the fact that he chose to have sex with another woman while he was supposed to still love me. Or maybe that's the point I've always been missing. Maybe he'd already stopped loving me.

"It's in the past," I tell him, slipping my hand away from his and edging away. "I'll just get those photos."

I go over to the sideboard at the other side of the room, my heart beating up a storm in my chest. I bend down, get Gigi's baby albums out, and take them over to Zeus.

I hand them to him, ensuring not to touch him again.

Zeus's touch always had a way of frazzling my brain, and it seems that some things don't die over time.

I sit back down on the sofa but a little further away this time.

I pick up my coffee and take a sip as he opens the book and starts to look through the pictures of Gigi's first minutes in the world.

"She had so much hair," he muses.

"Like you," I say, remembering his baby pictures.

He glances up at me and smiles that smile of his, and my chest constricts with long-ago hidden emotion.

"How much did she weigh?" he asks, looking through the pictures.

"Eight pounds."

His smile expands. "Big girl."

"She was all legs," I tell him. "Still is."

"She gets it from you." He nods at my jean-covered legs.

"Yeah, well, you're not exactly small," I infer.

He chuckles.

He goes quiet as he stares down at the pictures that Aunt Elle took of me holding Gigi not long after she was born.

"Elle was with you when you gave birth," he says, but it's not a question.

"Yes."

He closes the photo album and drives his fingers into his hair, exhaling a harsh breath. He tips his head to the side and looks at me. "I'm so fucking sorry that I wasn't there, Cam. That I haven't been here for the last five years."

"I don't know what to say, Zeus. You want me to say it's fine. It's not. But I managed."

"You must've hated me."

"You really want me to answer that?"

He moves his hands from his head. "The coward in

me wants to say no. But I deserve everything you want to throw my way."

"I . . . look, when we broke up . . . what you did, yeah, I hated you for that. Part of me still does. But it was five years ago—"

"Cam—"

"Just . . . let me finish, Zeus. It's in the past, and it doesn't matter anymore. But thinking, for all these years, that you abandoned Gigi, just walked away from her, yeah, I hated your guts. But . . . now, I know different. And I just need to know that you mean it when you say you want to be a part of her life."

"I do want to." His eyes fix on mine. "I want to know my daughter. I'm not going anywhere."

"Why are you back in New York?"

His eyes drift to the wall in front of him. His jaw tightening. "For a fight. I have training camp."

"So, you're still boxing?" I ask him.

Twelve months ago, Zeus had a big title match against Kaden Scott for the world heavyweight championship. Zeus was the favorite to win. He's currently undefeated with a total of twenty-one fights, all twenty-one wins by knockout.

I didn't watch it. I never watch Zeus's fights anymore. But, that same night, I saw on the news that Zeus and Kaden had gone eleven rounds. Zeus's longest fight.

They were both exhausted. The fight should've been stopped. It wasn't. Honestly, I wouldn't put it past Marcel, having had some influence on that.

Zeus got the advantage in the eleventh round and knocked Kaden to the floor with one uppercut hit.

Kaden went down. He got back up, but it was over, and Zeus was declared the winner.

When Zeus was doing his post-fight interview, Kaden collapsed in the ring.

Brain injury. There was a clot on his brain.

From what I read in the papers, Kaden was in a coma for thirty days. He had multiple surgeries to remove the clot. He suffered from a stroke. From what I last read, he was paralyzed down the right side of his body and had speech problems. He's currently still in the hospital, undergoing rehabilitation.

After the fight, Zeus disappeared from the public eye for twelve months. Not that the press or public blamed him for what had happened to Kaden. But I can understand why he went into hiding.

I heard some reports that Zeus would go to the hospital where Kaden was receiving treatment. I wasn't surprised, knowing Zeus.

Well, the Zeus I knew from five years ago. And irrespective of what he did to me, going by his reaction to finding out that he had a daughter, I would imagine it to be true.

Knowing all this, after I saw him last night, I did a Google search on him to see why he was here in New York. I had a gut feeling it was for a fight, and I was right. He's fighting Roman Dimitrov in twelve weeks.

I'd say I was shocked he was going to fight again, but I'm not. It's who Zeus is. Boxing is all he knows.

"I know what you're thinking," he says low.

I flash a look his way. "No, you don't."

"You're thinking I'm a bastard to fight after what

happened with Scott. You're also thinking that I'll be at training camp to intensively prep for this fight with Dimitrov, so I won't have time for Gigi."

"Aside from the fact that I can't believe you're fighting Dimitrov—the guy's a complete psycho—"

"I can take him, Cam," he cuts me off.

"And maybe lose a chunk of flesh in the process."

Dimitrov bit his last opponent on his neck when he was getting the better of him. Took a chunk out of him. The guy is a dog.

"He won't get near me," Zeus growls, sounding pissy that I'm even questioning him on this.

"Whatever, Zeus. Do what you want. You always have. But I know for a fact that you won't have time for Gigi in the lead up to this fight. And I'm not introducing you into her life now, only for you to disappear on her in a few weeks."

"What are you saying?"

"Maybe wait until the fight is over." I soften my tone. "Then, we'll introduce you into her life."

"No. I want to know my daughter now. I'll postpone the fight if I have to."

That does surprise me. But knowing he would do that for her makes me feel a little better about bringing him into her life.

"Won't that cause you problems?" I ask.

"Let me worry about that. Marcel set up the fight. And, with the way things stand with him and me right now, he's going to be lucky if he's still breathing when I'm finished with him."

"Okay, so you postpone the fight. It'll still have to happen at some point. You'll still be boxing. You'll still be spending inordinate amounts of time away from Gigi when you're training."

"You want me to quit?"

"I'm not asking you to do anything."

"Don't shy away from the truth, Cam. It's not you."

"Like I said, I don't want my daughter getting attached to you, for you to disappear on her." I know just how much it hurts, having Zeus in your life, and for him to one day be gone.

The look he throws my way sears right through me. "I won't disappear on her."

"You said those exact words to me," I toss back at him. "At the airport, the first time you left to go to the Olympics. 'I'm not gonna disappear on you, Dove,' " I say, imitating his voice.

"Jesus, Cam. I know I screwed up big time with us. And I hate that I did. I can't change that. But I can promise that I won't screw up with Gigi. But you can't ask me to quit boxing at the moment. I have to fight. I don't have a choice."

"Of course you don't." I laugh emptily. "Your bank account must've taken a hammering over the years with all the women you've been entertaining."

Jesus, I'm bitter. I don't know how many women there's been since me. But a week after Zeus broke up with me, he was photographed shopping with some model. I figured it was the one he'd cheated on me with. And I took it as his message to me to stay away.

His gaze snaps to mine. Eyes wide and angry. "I'm okay for money. But I have a family to support. A brother and sister in college. And, now, I have my daughter's future to secure. So, no, Cam, I can't stop fighting right now. The Dimitrov fight will bring in big money. I have to do it."

"And then you're done?"

He looks at me and slowly shakes his head. "I don't know."

"So, you want to come into my daughter's life and just be there when you can be?"

"Cam . . ."

"Don't *Cam* me. I know what it's like when you're training for a fight. It can take you away for months at a time."

"You're not being fair."

"No, you're not being fair. I won't have you hurting my daughter, Zeus."

"She's my daughter, too! And I've missed four years of her life because you didn't try hard enough to contact me!" he bellows so loud that, at first, it takes me aback, winds me. But then it incites me to levels of anger I didn't know existed within me until now.

I get to my feet. "Fuck. You. Zeus. You cheated on me. You slept with another woman. You left me. You broke up with me over the phone. You didn't even have the courtesy of saying it to my face. Then, you cut me off cold. Even blocked my e-mails, for fuck's sake! How was I supposed to contact you? I couldn't get near you to talk to you. I did the best I could. I spoke to the one person who did have access to you. It's not my fault he's a deceptive son of a bitch. What I did might not have been as good as what the almighty Zeus would have done, but I did what I could. And I have successfully raised *my* daughter for the past four years without you. I don't need you. And Gigi sure as hell doesn't."

I know what I'm saying is shitty and wrong. But I want to hurt him in this moment, just like he hurt me.

"Cam. Fuck. I'm sorry. I didn't mean it . . ." He gets to his feet, eyes bright with panic, and reaches for me.

I step away from his reach and protectively fold my arms around my chest. "Yes, you did. And, now, it's time for you to leave."

"No, please. Cam." He scrubs his hand over his head, fingers gripping the strands of hair. "I shouldn't have said that. I don't mean it, and you know I don't. My head is just all over the place. I just found out I've got a daughter, for Christ's sake. And I might not be thinking a hundred percent straight. But Gigi is my daughter, and I want to be a part of her life. I *need* to be a part of her life. And I swear to you and her that nothing will ever come in the way of my relationship with Gigi. I will never hurt her."

Chapter Seven

I STARE AT ZEUS, WAVERING between anger, and anguish, and the knowledge that I can't keep his daughter from him. It's not who I am. It's not in me to hurt someone that way. And keeping Gigi from him would only hurt her, and I will never hurt her.

I relax my hold on myself and exhale a breath.

"If you let her down, Zeus . . . I'll kill you myself."

"I won't let her down. I swear to God." He steps closer to me. So close that I can smell his aftershave. That same unfamiliar yet familiar scent.

"You changed your aftershave," I say. I know it's a stupid thing to say the instant the words are out of my mouth, but knowing that he wanted to erase me from his life, even down to this, bothers me. Hurts me.

"The old one reminded me of you," he says low.

Well, hell, if that doesn't sting.

I'm staring at his chest. I don't want him to see the emotion in my eyes right now.

"Well, I'm sorry to have been a bother. I guess it

must have been awkward, fucking other women with the scent of the last one all over you."

"Jesus, Cam. That's not what I meant, and you know it."

"Do I?" I make the error of looking up into his eyes. I know it's a mistake the second I do.

It's like dynamite being tossed onto an already raging fire between us.

Attraction explodes between us.

Zeus's eyes are burning for me in that way they used to, and it makes my soul ache. I feel a million things in this moment. Not one of them sensible or smart.

It reminds me of days long gone. Wanting each other was never a problem for us. Even in the early days of our relationship when we were taking things slow. I always knew Zeus wanted me.

Until he wanted other people.

And that is like a bucket of cold water over my head.

I step back and wrap my arms around myself. My heart is hammering in my chest. "Gigi will be home soon," I say, needing him to leave now. "It'd probably be better if you weren't here when she came home."

"Okay," he agrees. "But can I see her tomorrow?"

"Yes. I'll talk to her when she gets home. Let her know we'll be spending some time with a new friend tomorrow."

As I walk him to the door, I ask about his family, "How's your dad?"

"Still drunk." Zeus shrugs it off like it doesn't matter, but I know better. "I put him in rehab twice," he tells me. "It didn't stick either time. He doesn't want to get sober. He gave up on living a long time ago. Now, he's just drinking himself to the grave."

That makes me hurt for him.

Brett Kincaid has been an alcoholic ever since I've known Zeus. He's not a mean drunk. Just a useless one. He started drinking after Zeus's mom, Grace, died. And it steadily got worse—to the point where he quit working and basically stayed home, drinking, all day long. That was when Zeus took over, caring for his brothers and sister. He left school before graduation and got a day job in a meat factory. He kept up with boxing, doing more fights to make money, and somehow managed to make time for me as well.

It was when he got invited to represent America at the Olympics that life took a turn for the better for him. But it was also the start of the end of us. His boxing career took off. And I got left behind, battered and bruised, in the wake of his success.

"I'm really sorry to hear that," I tell him. "Knowing he's got a granddaughter might help," I add hopefully.

"Yeah, maybe." But he doesn't sound convinced.

"How's Ares doing?" I ask as we reach the door.

He was at Penn State. Starting quarterback for the Lions.

Zeus smiles, probably the first real smile that I've seen on him since he walked back into my life last night. "He got drafted by the Giants. First pick. He's in his second season with them."

"Wow. That's amazing," I say, and I mean it. I always liked Ares. "How about the twins?"

"Lo's in his third year at Penn State. He followed Ares there. And Missy's in her third year at Dartmouth."

Lo and Missy are Zeus's nicknames for Apollo and Artemis.

"I'm not surprised they went to separate universities. Lo and Missy always wanted their independence from each other." I snicker.

"Yeah." Zeus chuckles. "They definitely fight less now that they live apart."

"That's great though," I tell him as I open the door to let him leave. "It sounds like they're all doing really well. You must be proud."

"Yeah, I am."

He walks outside, and I stand by the door, holding it.

"What will you tell them about Gigi?" I ask him.

"The truth."

"They're going to hate me."

"They're going to hate Marcel. Well, not that they particularly like him anyway. Not many people do."

"You included."

"Yep."

"Why stay with him all these years if he's such a bastard?"

"Because he brings in the best fights. And he's only a bastard to other people. Not to me. Well"—he lets out a humorless laugh—"or so I thought."

"Why do you think he did it? Lied to both of us?"

He briefly closes his eyes and exhales a harsh breath before staring back at me. "For the reason Marcel does everything—money."

"I don't understand."

"I was on the rise. I was set to make him a lot of money, which I have. But he always saw you as a threat to ‘my success’—as he called it. He was always on my back, saying that you were an unnecessary distraction.”

Ouch.

“Unnecessary. Nice.”

He winces. “Sorry.”

“Don’t be. I guess it explains why . . . well, whatever. It doesn’t matter now anyway.”

He’s staring at me. His expression unreadable. “Cam—”

“So, I was a distraction, and what? He thought Gigi would have been an even bigger distraction,” I cut him off before he can say something that I really don’t want to hear.

“Yeah.” He shrugs. “I guess he thought that, if I knew you were pregnant, my focus would have been on you and the baby. Not boxing. Which it absolutely would’ve been. Marcel wouldn’t have wanted that. He sees the fighters he manages and promotes as investments. He wanted a return on me, which he got.”

“What will you do . . . about Marcel?”

I watch as his hands flex at his sides.

“Something.”

“Zeus, please don’t do anything stupid.”

“I won’t.” He nods.

But the look in his eyes doesn’t make me fully believe him.

“There’s something else . . .” I say.

“You’re seeing someone?” he says roughly, making my spine straighten like I’ve just been hit with a cattle prod.

“What? Where in the hell did that come from?”

He grits his teeth, holding my eyes. “I don’t want

another guy coming between me getting to know my daughter, Cam."

I frown. "No one will be interfering with you getting to know your daughter, Zeus."

He nods. "So . . . is there a guy?"

Rich.

I shift on my feet and swallow. "Yes. No. Kind of. It's not serious," I tell him. Why I tell him that it's not serious with Rich, I have no clue. That incites me to add, "Not that it's any of your business."

His jaw tightens. He can't hide his anger from me. I just don't get why he is angry.

"If he's around Gigi, then it is my business."

Ah, so that's why.

"Gigi doesn't know that Rich and I are seeing each other. She thinks he's just a guy I work with."

"At the club?"

"No. The station. He's a police officer. I work in admin at Aunt Elle's precinct during the day. I only work at the club on weekends."

"Jesus, Cam. You work two jobs?"

"Gigi's always well cared for," I state defensively.

"That's not what I'm worried about. I'm talking about you working two jobs to earn money to care for our kid."

"I'm fine for money. The job at the station gives me enough for us to live comfortably. Living here with Aunt Elle takes off the pressure. I only dance at the club . . . well, for me, so I don't forget how to dance. And the extra money I earn there, I'm saving for when Gigi's older."

"Well, you don't need to now. I'll be giving you all

the money you need for Gigi. So, you can quit both jobs."

"I'm not quitting my job!" I exclaim.

His eyes narrow. "Why? So that you can keep on seeing your secret boyfriend?"

My brows slam angrily together. "Rich isn't my boyfriend. And I'm not quitting my job because I don't need you taking care of me." *Asshole*, I silently add at the end.

"Well, I'm giving you money either way because I take care of what's mine."

"I'm not yours," I fire back at him.

He steps forward. "No. But Gigi is. And you're her mother."

I step back and fold my arms over my chest. "Whatever. I'm not quitting my job."

He sighs heavily. "Do what you want, Cam. Just make sure that Deputy Dick doesn't get in my way, and then we won't have any problems."

"Deputy Dick? Jesus, Zeus. Childish much? And, for your information, he's not a deputy."

"Traffic cop? Thought so."

"He's a police officer," I snap. "God, why are you being such an asshole about this?"

His face instantly clears, and he steps away.

I hate the way he can just wipe emotion away like it was never there. Like it never mattered.

"You're right. I am being a dick. It won't happen again. What time should I be here tomorrow?"

I loosen my arms, letting some of the tension go from them.

"Eleven a.m. We can take Gigi out to the park. She

loves it there. I'll come with you this time and probably the next few times. Afterward, I won't come along. It's just that she doesn't know you right now, and—"

"You don't have to explain, Cam. I'm glad you'll be there."

Glad. I'm not really sure how to take that.

He steps off the porch. "So, I'll see you tomorrow at eleven."

"Yeah, just . . ."

"Just what?"

"There's something else I wanted to ask."

"Hit me with it."

"You're in the public eye. I don't want that for Gigi."

"Don't worry. I'll keep her protected."

"Okay." I breathe my relief. "Thank you."

"Not necessary. I'll see you tomorrow, Cam." He turns and starts to walk down the path.

I watch him leave, this strange clutching feeling in my chest.

"Zeus?" I call.

He stops immediately and turns around to me.

I walk to the edge of the porch. "Can I ask you something else?"

He moves a few steps back toward me. "You can ask me anything."

I wrap my hand around the wooden porch post, leaning my hip against it. "Why did you come today? I thought it was because of Gigi, but you didn't know about her."

Zeus pushes his hands into his pockets. His eyes sweep the ground before they come back to rest on mine, strong and focused but also resigned. He exhales a breath and parts his lips. "For you. I came for you, Dove."

Then, without another word, he turns and walks away.

And I let him.

Chapter Eight

GOD, WHAT A MESS.

All these years, Zeus had no clue that Gigi existed.

Aunt Elle was suspicious at first when I told her that Zeus knew nothing about me being pregnant and that Marcel had lied to both me and Zeus.

She said, "Just because Zeus said it doesn't make it true."

I questioned why he would have lied.

And she shrugged and said, "Why does anyone lie?"

I hadn't even considered it, to be honest.

But I guess Aunt Elle deals with liars every single day, that it's part of her makeup now to be suspicious of people.

I could tell Zeus wasn't lying. His reaction alone when he realized he had a daughter wasn't something you could fake.

I spent all these years hating him for walking away from Gigi, and now, I know the truth . . . that he didn't abandon her. I don't know how to feel.

He cheated on me. That fact hasn't changed.

And, now, it's all I've got left to hold on to, to keep my anger and resentment alive for him.

Because seeing Zeus after all this time has rattled my emotions. It always was impossible for me to be around him and not feel something.

And, after his parting words yesterday, I have to keep him at arm's length.

"I came for you."

I don't know exactly what he meant by that. What he wanted from me. Well, whatever it was, I don't intend to find out.

Zeus broke my heart, and I won't let him do it again.

He's here for Gigi now, and that's fine. Well, it's not fine. It's hard.

It feels difficult that she's going to have another parent now. I've been her only one for so long. And, as much as I'm glad that she's going to have her father, it's still scary for me that, going forward, I'm going to have to share her with Zeus.

I'm dressed and ready and sipping on a cup of coffee, trying to steady my jittery nerves before he gets here.

Gigi's upstairs, getting dressed.

I told her yesterday that we were going out to the park with an old friend of Mommy's. And, being the kid she is, she heard the word *park*, and nothing else registered. To her, it's no big deal.

But it's everything.

And I don't know if I'm handling this whole situation right.

If there's a certain way I should be doing things.

Maybe I'm getting it wrong, not telling Gigi right

away that Zeus is her father. I just don't want to confuse or upset her. I think, if she at least knows him before I drop the bombshell, it might make things easier.

I hope.

Zeus is easy to fall in love with.

I learned that the hard way.

I just pray that Gigi never has to experience what it's like to lose Zeus.

Aunt Elle wanders into the kitchen, ready for work. "You look pretty," she says.

I stare down at my outfit.

I'm wearing skinny jeans and a chunky white knit top with thigh-high brown boots. I curled my hair, and I'm wearing makeup. I wouldn't usually make this much of an effort to take Gigi to the park, but he is my ex, who left me for another woman, and I refuse to look shitty around him.

"Too much?" I ask.

"Perfect." She winks.

I grab a cup, pour her some coffee, and hand it to her. No need to ask Aunt Elle if she wants one. Her blood type is caffeine.

"Where's Gigi?" she asks.

"Upstairs, getting dressed. She insisted on dressing herself," I tell Aunt Elle.

She raises her brows. "Should be interesting."

Gigi's style can be a little flamboyant when she's allowed to dress herself.

"I'm actually looking forward to seeing what she wears." I chuckle.

"You ready for today?"

"Nope."

"It's going to be fine, Cam."

"I don't know." I sigh.

"Cam, he screwed you over, and I hate him for it. But, if you believe he knew nothing about you being pregnant, then I believe him. And, after thinking about it, it does makes sense. Family is important to Zeus. Fidelity, not so much. But his family is everything to him. He would do anything for those brothers and that sister of his. Gigi's his blood. He's not going to hurt her."

"Yeah, you're right."

"I'm always right." She grins, drains her coffee, and puts her cup down in the sink. "I'm heading into the station. But I can wait to leave if you want me to hang around until Zeus arrives."

"No, you head off. I'll be fine."

I hear the telltale thud of Gigi coming down the stairs. For a dancer who's light on her feet, she sure is like an elephant on those steps.

"Mommy?" she calls.

"Kitchen," I call back.

With a smile on my face, I watch her through the open doorway as she wanders toward me.

She's wearing black leggings with skulls on them, which were part of last year's Halloween costume. A gray *My Little Pony* T-shirt, denim jacket, and her brown fur-lined boots. And, to finish the ensemble, a bright blue tutu, which was part of her costume from her last dance recital.

She actually looks cool as hell.

"Well, look at you, Gigi girl," Aunt Elle says when she enters the kitchen.

"You *wike* my clothes, Granny Elle?"

Aunt Elle picks her up and kisses her cheek. "I love them. You look beautiful." She lowers Gigi to her feet. "Right, Granny Elle's going to work. You have a good time today, Gigi girl."

Aunt Elle stops and kisses me on the cheek. "Breathe," she whispers to me. "It will be fine. And, remember, I know how to dispose of a body without it ever being found."

I meet her twinkling eyes and chuckle. "Love you," I tell her.

"Love you, too. And love my Gigi girl." She blows Gigi a kiss and then walks out of the kitchen.

I turn to Gigi as Aunt Elle leaves. "You want me to do your hair?" I ask Gigi.

"No. Want to wear it down."

"Have you brushed it?" I already know the answer to that question.

"I's get the brush," she sings and skips out of the kitchen. A few minutes later, she returns with the brush and her favorite headband that has Disney princesses on it. "Can you put this on, Mommy?"

"Sure, baby." I brush her long hair out. Then, I move in front of her and fix the headband in place. I lean down and place a kiss on the tip of her nose. "Pretty girl," I tell her.

She presses her hands to my cheeks. "Not as *pwetty* as you, Mommy."

"No way!" I exclaim. "You're way prettier than Mommy."

She grins at me.

Jesus, I love her so much, it hurts sometimes.

I just pray to God that Zeus doesn't hurt her.

I glance at the clock on the wall. Ten fifty-five. I told him to be here at eleven. He'd better not be late. Zeus and being on time didn't always have the best relationship.

A minute later, the doorbell rings.

And my heart gallops off into a race.

I open the door.

Zeus is standing there, looking as handsome as ever in blue jeans and a black sweater.

"Hi," I say.

"Hey, Cam." His eyes hold mine for a beat before coming down to Gigi. "Hey, Gigi." He smiles widely at her. "You look really pretty today. Is that a tutu?"

"Gigi dressed herself today," I tell him.

"Well, I think you did a great job. These are for you." He brings his hand from behind his back. He's holding a large gift bag and a bunch of daisies that are all wrapped up and look like they came from a florist.

"You got me a *pwesent*? And flowers? But it's not my birthday."

I see the pain that flickers across his countenance, and I just know he's thinking about the four birthdays that he's already missed.

"I know, but I wanted to get you a gift. I hope that's okay?" His question is more for me than Gigi.

I give him a small nod, telling him it's fine, and his expression relaxes.

"Say thank you, Gigi."

"Thank you."

"And I got these for you." He pulls out from behind

his back a bunch of oriental lilies, my favorite flower, and hands them to me.

I blankly stare down at them, my heart racing in my chest.

"You don't like them anymore?" His face falls.

"No. I mean, yes. It's just . . ." I glance down at Gigi and then back to Zeus. "You don't have to bring me flowers."

"I know I don't. I wanted to."

"I just don't think it's *appropriate*," I whisper that last word.

His brows furrow with a flash of anger in his eyes; if I didn't know him as well as I do, I would have missed it.

"It's just a gift, Dove."

"Dove?" Gigi says, sounding confused.

"It's a nickname I used to call your mom," Zeus explains to her.

"You knew my mom before you was our new mailman?"

"Gigi, this is Zeus. The friend I was telling you about."

Gigi stares at me puzzled. "Your friend is our new mailman?"

Me and my big, stupid mouth.

"Oh. Well, um, I . . . I . . ." I'm faltering.

"I was your new mailman." Zeus steps in for me, crouching down in front of Gigi so that he's eye-level with her. "But I'm not very good at it, so your old mailman is coming back."

"Oh, that's sad for you. But I'm happy that Burt's back, so he can tell me more jokes."

Zeus's lip lifts at the corner. "I know I'm not your mailman anymore, but I'd like to be your friend, if that's okay with you?"

Gigi's big blue eyes blink up at me, looking for confirmation that it's okay.

"It's okay, Gigi."

"Okay, we can be friends." She steps a little closer to him and whispers, "Just so you know, I'm an awesome *fwiend* to have."

Zeus chuckles. "I bet you are."

"What's your name?" she asks even though I told her it not one minute ago. "'Cause, if we *fwiends*, I has to know your name."

"Zeus Kincaid." He holds his hand out to her, and she puts her little hand in his. "It's nice to meet you."

"*Zweus* is a funny name." The way she says his name is the cutest thing ever.

Still, the parent in me has to call her out for saying his name is funny. "Gigi, that's not a nice thing to say."

"Sorry," she says to Zeus, lowering her eyes and pulling her hand from his, retreating back to my side.

"It's fine." He smiles warmly at her. "It is a funny name. Not pretty like yours. But you know, Gigi, I was named after a god."

Her eyes widen. "You know God's name?" she says with awe.

Zeus chuckles. "Not God's name. Zeus was a Greek god. The god of the sky. He controlled thunder and lightning."

"I's scared of thunder and lightning."

"Well then, I'll protect you from them." He winks at her before rising to stand.

"So, shall we get going then?" I say. "Let's put these inside," I tell Gigi, taking the flowers and present from her.

"Can I open it now?" she asks.

"Sure," I tell her.

She rips the paper off, handing it to me, and lets out a shriek. "Mommy, look! It's the Magical Princess Twilight Sparkle!" She hugs it to her chest.

She's shrieking because she's been desperate for one. But, with a price tag of a hundred dollars, it's a tad out of my budget.

"That's a really expensive toy," I say to Zeus, my brows lifting.

He just shrugs. "The lady in the shop said it's the big toy this year."

And didn't she just see him coming?

I smile at his generosity. "It's really kind of you," I tell him. "Say thank you to Zeus, Gigi."

"Thank you, *Zweus*!" Gigi runs at him and wraps her arms around his leg, hugging him.

The look on his face makes my heart constrict in my chest. I watch as his eyes fill with that level of emotion that only your child can make you feel.

He places his hand on her head and clears his throat. "You're welcome, Gigi." His voice sounds like gravel.

Gigi lets go of him, her expression one of absolute joy. "Can I take it to the park with me, Mommy?"

"I don't know. It's an expensive toy, Gigi."

"I be careful, I *pwomise. Pwease*, Mommy." She begs with those gorgeous eyes of hers.

"How about this? You can take it with you. But,

when we reach the park, Princess Twilight Sparkle will stay with Mommy until you're done playing."

"Yay! Mommy, you da best!" She bounces on the spot.

"Let me just put these inside"—I gesture to the flowers—"and then we can get going."

I go inside, leaving Gigi on the porch with Zeus. I quickly fill the sink with water, sitting the flowers in it. I'll put them in vases when I get back.

I grab my bag and my and Gigi's jackets.

When I get back on the porch, Gigi and Zeus are sitting on a step, and she's giving Zeus a full lowdown on all the *My Little Pony* character names. He's intently staring at her, hanging on every word she's saying.

I feel an ache in my chest for him because he's missed out on four years with her.

"Ready?" I say.

They both turn, and Zeus gets to his feet. Gigi hops up.

"Whereabouts is the park?" Zeus asks me.

"It's a fifteen-minute walk. But we can drive there if you want. I was thinking we could get some lunch afterward at Gigi's favorite diner, if you want?" I want them to have a decent amount of time together.

"Sounds perfect." He smiles wide. "I can drive us there. I've got a car."

"Gigi needs a car seat," I tell him.

"All covered." He walks off our porch and down the garden path, toward an Audi A7. "Rental car. I had them put in a car seat."

I warm at the knowledge that he thought to do that.

Gigi skips over to his car. He opens the back passenger door, letting her in.

I watch with amusement as he struggles to fasten her into the car seat.

"It's easy, Zeus. That *stwap* goes over here and then *cwicks* in there."

"You want me to do it?" I offer.

"No. I got it."

"You sure?"

"Yep."

I hear a grumble and a grunt. Then, finally, a click.

"Yay! Good job, *Zweus*! You dids it!" Gigi claps, and I laugh.

The look I get from Zeus is one of amusement.

"You need a college degree to fasten that thing."

I nod in agreement.

I climb in the passenger side and buckle myself in.

Zeus gets in. I give him directions to the park, and then we're off.

"Where are you staying?" I ask him.

He glances at me. "I was staying with Ares at his place in New York. But since . . ." He moves his eyes in Gigi's direction. "I wanted to be closer, so I'm at the Travelodge in Manhasset."

I laugh softly and shake my head.

"What?" He gives me a puzzled look.

"You're driving an Audi A7 but staying in a Travelodge. You do know there's a nice hotel not far from the marina."

"I don't need a nice hotel, Cam. It's just a place to sleep and shower. I do need a safe car for Gigi to ride in, and this is one of the best."

Well, if that doesn't put me in my place in the best kind of way.

Zeus has always been a basic kind of guy. Material things have never really mattered to him.

People who he loves are what matter to Zeus.

That's what made it hurt all the more when he just disregarded me without a second thought.

Gigi starts talking in the backseat, telling Zeus that we're passing by her friend's house, and she doesn't stop commanding his attention. And he thoughtfully listens to her, taking it all in.

I half-listen to her—partly because I already know everything she's saying, but also because being in this car with him is assaulting me with the hundreds of memories of time spent in the old Chevy truck that Zeus used to drive.

When my eyes fix on his strong hands on the steering wheel, my memories move off into a whole other territory, and I feel myself flush.

It's like he can read my thoughts. His eyes turn to mine and hold for a fraction of a second, but the heat in his eyes is unmistakable.

"I came for you."

I avert my eyes and stare out the passenger window, my heart beating out of my chest.

Chapter Nine

THERE ARE A FEW kids at the park when we arrive. But Gigi doesn't go over to them. She heads straight for the empty swings, and Zeus follows behind her because she wants him to push her on one.

I follow, hugging Princess Twilight Sparkle to my chest, as Gigi wouldn't leave her in the car. She said she'd get lonely there without us.

I recognize some of the parents in the park from Gigi's school. I wave but don't go over to talk to them like I normally would, as I don't want to have to answer awkward questions about Zeus, and I opt to take a seat on the bench near the swings.

He puts on a ball cap that he pulled out of the glove box. "Just in case," he told me.

I am hoping they don't recognize him, as I don't want people asking why he's here with me and Gigi. But I know it's wishful thinking on my part. Zeus stands out. With his huge height and massive frame, he's unmissable. He also has an aura about him that just attracts people to him. And it doesn't help that he's incredibly good-looking.

Well, it doesn't help me at the moment.

It's easy to remember all the reasons I fell in love with this guy and forget all the reasons we're not together now.

I watch him with Gigi. She's on the swing, and he's pushing her.

She's giggling and saying, "Higher, *Zweus*! Higher!"

"Not too high, Gigi," the concerned parent in me calls over.

Zeus nods at me, telling me that he's got it. Not in a crappy way. More of a trust-me way.

And I'm going to have to trust him with my—*our* daughter. It's just hard. I've been parenting Gigi alone for the last four years. It's going to be hard, letting him have a say. But I have to. And this is the start of it.

"Slide now, *Zweus*!" Gigi jumps off the swing before it stops moving, giving me anxiety. She runs over to the slide, which is closer to the parents.

I can see the way they're looking at him, especially one of the dads, like he recognizes Zeus.

And, if they haven't figured out who he is, then they will from Gigi calling out Zeus's name.

It's not your average name.

I watch as they talk among themselves. The dad is sliding looks in Zeus's direction as he follows Gigi around, moving from the slide to the merry-go-round.

Bringing us here was probably poor judgment on my part. I forgot how well known he is now. But then where can we go and not risk him being recognized?

This is going to be the hard part. Keeping who Zeus is to Gigi under wraps until it's time for us to tell her. But I have a feeling that telling Gigi that Zeus is her dad will have to come an awful lot sooner than I would prefer.

I get up from the bench and walk over to them at the merry-go-round.

When I reach Zeus, who is laughing at something Gigi just said as she whizzes around while he spins her, I step close to him and say, "You've been made." I jerk my head in the direction of the parents.

"Yeah. I figured." He exhales.

"You want to leave?"

He shakes his head, meeting my eyes. "No. I want to stay here until Gigi's ready to leave."

"Oh, well, in that case, we'll be here all day. Right, Gigi girl?" I say, and she grins.

"I loves the park!" she squeals as she spins past us. "Keep spinning, *Zweus*! Faster!"

"Not too fast, or you'll throw up. Remember last time?"

"I puked," she says to Zeus, a grim expression on her face. "I had ice *cweam* and had Granny Elle spin me fast."

"Blue bubblegum ice cream," I tell him. "It wasn't a pretty sight."

He laughs deep, a rumble in his chest. "Glad I missed it," he says. Then, a flash of pain crosses his brow at his own words.

I want to say something to make him feel better, but I don't know what.

And then we're interrupted by a voice behind us.

"Hey, man."

Zeus and I turn to the voice, finding the dad who was eyeballing Zeus.

"Sorry to bother you . . . but are you Zeus Kincaid?"

Zeus smiles. It's forced. But you'd have to know him as well as I do to know that.

"Yeah," he says.

The guy's expression brightens. "I thought so. God, man, I can't believe it. I'm a big fan. I used to box when I was younger—nothing like you, of course. You're amazing."

"Thanks. I appreciate it," Zeus says.

"Would it be okay if I got a picture with you?"

I just look at Zeus. You can tell he doesn't want to. But I know what he's going to say.

He glances back at Gigi, who's waiting on the merry-go-round, which has slowed to a stop. She has a curious expression on her face.

"I'll just be a sec, okay?"

She nods but doesn't say anything.

The guy digs his cell out of his pocket and holds it out to me. "Would you mind?"

I take the phone and snap the photo. Then, I hand the phone back to him.

"Thanks," he says to me. "Sorry to interrupt," he says to us all. "And good luck with the Dimitrov fight," he tells Zeus. "Not that you'll need it. I reckon five rounds, most."

"Thanks, man," Zeus says to him. Then, he turns back to Gigi. "Sorry about that, Gigi. Right, you want me to keep spinning you, or are we going on something else?"

She doesn't answer. She's staring at him, her head cocked to the side, like she does when she's trying to work something out.

For a split second, my heart stops as I worry that she's figured out he's her dad, which is crazy. There's no way she'd be able to figure that out. Right?

"Why dids that man want to take picture with you, *Zweus*?"

"Well . . ." He seems to be struggling with how to answer.

"Zeus has a job that means he's sometimes on TV," I tell her.

"*Wike* Princess Twilight Sparkle?"

"Kind of but different," I answer.

"Different how?" she asks, craning her head to look up at Zeus.

He crouches down in front of her, so he's eye-level. "Well, I'm a boxer, Gigi."

Her brows come together. "But I's thought you were a mailman?"

His lip comes out at the corner, forming his trademark half-smile. "That was my other job. But my main job is boxing."

"So . . . you's a box?"

Zeus rumbles out a laugh. "A boxer—a fighter," he explains to her.

"Fighting's bad." She frowns. "Mommy always tells me that."

"Your mom's right; fighting is bad, Gigi. But there are some instances when it's okay."

"*Wike*?"

"Well, when it's a sport, like boxing is. I put on

gloves and get in a boxing ring to fight against another boxer. There's a referee to make sure we're okay. And medics are on standby in case one of us gets hurt."

"You get hurt?" Her eyes widen, and the concern on her face tugs at my chest.

"No," he tells her, his expression softening. "I'm the best. And, when you're the best like me, no one gets close enough to hurt you."

Those words echo in my mind, and I believe them down to my very core.

I can't imagine anyone ever hurting Zeus. And I don't mean just physically.

Chapter Ten

WE STAYED IN THE park for another hour, and no one bothered Zeus for a picture again, which was good. We're back in his car now and on our way to Landmark Diner, which is Gigi's favorite place to eat, as she loves their pancakes.

She also seems to really like Zeus. She's been soaking up attention all morning. He's totally gone for her. I can see it in his eyes. But then Gigi is easy to love. She gets that trait from her father.

Watching Zeus with Gigi—something I never thought I'd see—makes me happy for her. That she finally has her father in her life even if she doesn't exactly know yet who he is.

But there's this permanent ache in my chest. I think it's the what-if ache. What if Zeus had never cheated on me and dumped me? We'd have been a family. Together for all this time.

But it's stupid to think about what-ifs. It gets you nowhere but to Sad Town.

Life happens the way it's meant to. And I was never supposed to be with Zeus for life.

I might have thought that he was the love of my life. And I can't deny that I still have feelings for him. He's Gigi's father and my first love, so I'm always going to have an emotional attachment to him. It makes sense.

But, beyond that, there's nothing more.

Zeus and I were over a long time ago.

"This the place?" Zeus checks as he pulls into the diner's parking lot.

"Yep. This is it."

"Looks nice," he comments as he parks the car in a space.

"It's my *favowite*," Gigi tells him for the tenth time.

He smiles at her in the rearview mirror.

Gigi insists on unbuckling herself. I notice Zeus doesn't put on his ball cap this time. Maybe because it didn't help him go unrecognized the last time.

Zeus gets out of the car, and I do the same. He opens the door for Gigi. She clambers out of the car with Princess Twilight Sparkle under her arm.

We all start to walk toward the diner. Gigi and Zeus are in front, and I'm just a little ways behind them.

"You gonna have pancakes, *Zweus*?" Gigi asks him.

"They make the best pancakes here, right?"

"Yep." She nods.

"Then, I'm having pancakes."

Then, she does something unexpected. She reaches up and takes hold of Zeus's hand.

His step falters. I watch him as he stares down at her tiny hand in his.

His eyes swing back to me.

The look on his face slays me, and for a second, I feel like I might burst into tears.

Those striking blue eyes of his are glittering with emotion.

I give him a tremulous smile. It's all I can manage.

And Gigi has no idea what such a small action means to that huge man beside her.

Gigi tugs on his hand. "Come on, *Zweus*. Pancakes!"

He bites down a smile and keeps moving with her into the diner.

I pick my heart up off the floor and walk through the door that Zeus is holding open for me.

"Thanks." I smile at him.

Gigi's already running over to a booth and climbing in it. She settles Princess Twilight Sparkle on her left side.

I take a seat across from her.

Zeus hesitates, seeming unsure of where to sit. But Gigi makes the decision for him.

"Sit here, *Zweus*." She pats the seat beside her.

He slides into the booth. His long legs bump into mine under the table.

My eyes flash up to his. Just even the touch of his jean-clad leg has heat racing up my skin.

"Sorry," he says, but his eyes don't look like he means it.

He shifts his legs to the side, so they're stretched just outside the booth.

"Hey, Miss Gigi, Cam," Megan, one of the waitresses, says, coming over to us.

We know everyone in here pretty well, as we're here often.

I see her steps falter as she spots Zeus sitting there. I watch as her eyes rake over Zeus, and I don't like the feeling it leaves in my stomach.

"Hi, Megan." Gigi beams at her. "You got me a picture to color?"

"Of course." Megan hands her one of the pictures and crayons that the diner provides to keep the kids entertained.

"And who's this?" Megan asks, her eyes on Zeus, a flirtatious edge to her expression that has me frowning.

"This is *Zweus*," Gigi volunteers up the information. "He's an old *fwiend* of Mommy's, and he's my new *fwiend*. And he's a box." She gives a toothy grin.

Zeus chuckles.

"Not a box, Gigi. A boxer," I remind her.

"Oh, yeah. I's forgot."

"Zeus Kincaid." Megan tips her head in an unmistakably flirtatious manner, a smile touching her lips. "The boxer."

"That's me," he says, grinning at her.

I have the sudden urge to kick him under the table.

Megan is pretty. Really pretty. A few years younger than me. Platinum-blonde hair. Has a bust size I'd kill for. She's nice. And I like her; I do. But, right now, I'm not liking so much the way she's looking at Zeus. Or the smile he's currently giving her in return.

I recognize that look on his face. He used to look at me that way when he was getting ready to disengage my clothes from me.

Something bitter twists in my gut.

He's supposed to be spending time getting to know his daughter, not flirting with the waitress.

Yeah, sure, Cam, that's the only reason you're all of a sudden feeling stabby.

"I know who you are. My brother's a big fan of yours," she says, smiling coyly at him, twirling her blonde hair around her finger. "He's gonna be real jealous that I've met you."

"I can sign an autograph for him if you'd like?" Zeus says to her.

"Wow. Really? He'd love that."

Of course, Zeus isn't keen on taking a picture with the nice dad in the park, but he has no problem with signing an autograph for the pretty waitress.

Megan tears off a piece of paper from her order pad and hands it to him along with her pen. She leans forward and rests her hand on the back of the seat behind him, and my eyes zero in on the action.

"And, if you want to write down your digits, too, I know someone else who would like that."

I see as she lightly brushes her fingers over his shoulder before moving back.

What?

Openly flirting in front of my kid. She doesn't know that Zeus and I aren't together, and she's just hitting on him like that.

Okay, I officially hate Megan.

I don't even bother to check out Zeus's reaction. He's probably loving the attention. And, if I see that, I might throw this napkin holder at him and grab Gigi's hand to take her out of here.

"Can we please order now?" I snap, and I'm not even sorry.

"Oh. Yeah, of course. Sorry." Megan says, not even seeming bothered.

I hear Zeus chuckle low, and I refuse to look at him or the piece of paper he's currently scribbling on to see if he's giving Megan his number as well.

I'm not looking. Definitely not.

I stare down at my menu, burning a hole in it.

"What can I get you guys to drink?" Megan asks.

"Coffee," I say without even looking up at her or waiting for Gigi to order first, and I feel like an ass.

I'm acting like a bad mom. And I hate that it's because of Zeus. Or rather my jealousy over Zeus.

Crap.

I glance up at Gigi, and thankfully, she has no clue that her mom is currently acting like a jealous shrew.

"What would you like to drink, Gigi girl?" I softly ask her.

"Milk, *pwease*," she says without looking up from her picture.

I glance at Megan to make sure she got that, and her writing on her pad tells me that she did.

"I'll have a coffee," Zeus rumbles out.

"Two coffees and a milk. Be right back with those."

Megan walks away, and I can't help but look at Zeus to see if he's watching her leave.

He's not. He's watching me. With something akin to amusement in his eyes.

And it pisses me off.

I frown at him. And you know what the bastard does?

He smiles at me.

"You *wike* my picture, *Zweus*?" Gigi asks him.

He pulls his eyes from me to look at her picture. "It's really good, Gigi. Do you like coloring?"

"S'okay," she says. Typical four-year-old response. "Yellow's my *favowite* color. Then, pink. Purple. And blue. What's your favorite color?" she asks him.

"Yellow," he says.

I know he's fibbing because green is his favorite color. Or it used to be.

"Same as me!" Gigi beams at him.

He smiles. "Same as you," he echoes.

Then, Megan Flirty McFlirterson appears back at our table with our drinks.

"Milk for Miss Gigi." She puts it on the table in front of Gigi, who immediately picks it up and has a drink.

"Coffee for Cam." She smiles at me as she puts it down in front of me.

I don't even bother to smile back. I think her behavior has been really inappropriate, asking for Zeus's number. I should complain to her boss.

"And coffee for Zeus." She puts down a small jug of creamer between Zeus and me.

I pick it up, knowing Zeus takes his coffee black and pour some into mine.

Then, because I'm feeling bitchy, I offer it to him.

He frowns. "I don't take creamer," he says roughly.

"Oh, yeah. I forgot."

His brow comes up. "You didn't forget yesterday when you made me a coffee."

Shit. Crap. And double shit.

I have nothing, so I ignore him and turn to Megan. "We're ready to order now."

I know Zeus hasn't even had a chance to look at the menu. But I'm not in the mood for playing nice right now. And Gigi knows everything on the menu here and has already decided what she's having, which will be—"I's have the cookies and *cweam* pancakes, *pwease*," Gigi says, taking the words right out of my head.

"What would you like, Zeus?" Megan asks him, a flirtatious lilt to her voice.

If he says her, I'm going to throat-punch him.

I'm not normally a violent person, but I'm feeling all kinds of ragey right now.

Zeus turns to Gigi. "What do you recommend I have?"

She looks up from her coloring to him. "Same as me. They da best."

He glances at Megan. "I'll have the same as Gigi, just double up the order for me."

"Growing guy, huh?" She simpers.

"I'm already grown," he says.

Her eyes flash to his huge biceps and then to his face. "Yes, you are," she says, biting the edge of her lip.

Right. I'm done.

"Blueberry pancakes for me," I say in a hard tone. "And send them with a different waitress."

Megan's eyes flash to mine. I stare hard at her. Her face reddens. Then, she gives me a look of apology, nods, and scurries off.

"You still have it, huh?" Zeus murmurs, seemingly nonplussed.

"What?" My voice is a quiet bite.

"A jealous streak."

My memory flies back to all those jealous moments I had over women flirting with him. He never once did anything wrong.

Until he did.

"I'm not jealous," I hiss, furious. "But we're also in a diner, not a bar. And my daughter is here."

Zeus actually has the good grace to look guilty. "I'm sorry. I wasn't trying to—"

"Forget it," I cut him off.

The atmosphere at the table is awful, so I break it by asking Gigi about her picture. It's the only thing I can think of to say. My brain's too full of angry barbs that I want to fire at Zeus at the moment.

"Cam," a recognizable voice says from beside me.

"Hey," I say, turning my head to see Rich standing there in his uniform.

"What are you doing here?" I ask nicely.

"Just picking up an order for me and some of the guys at the station. Hey, Gigi." He gives her a wave.

"Hi, Rich." She waves back, smiling.

At the mention of Rich's name, I see Zeus stiffen in my peripheral. If we hadn't just had the Megan situation, then I would feel awkward about Rich being here. Now, not so much.

Rich's eyes curiously go to Zeus, recognition sparking in them.

Zeus is openly glaring at him.

Ah, crap.

Okay, so maybe I am feeling a little uncomfortable.

Knowing I have to introduce them, I say, "Rich, this is Zeus Kincaid. Zeus, this is Rich Hastings."

"I know who you are," Rich says to Zeus, putting a hand out to shake Zeus's. "I'm a big fan."

Zeus looks at his outstretched hand like it's smeared with the Ebola virus, and then he somewhat reluctantly shakes his hand. Hard, if going by the way Rich flexes his fingers after their handshake.

"Always good to meet a fan," Zeus says. And I'm pretty sure I detect sarcasm in his voice.

"So, how do you guys know each other?" Rich asks.

"*Zweus* is an old friend of Mommy's," Gigi helpfully says.

"We went to school together," I clarify, leaving out the part that he was my first love, my first everything. "Zeus is in town, so we're just catching up."

"What brings you to Port Washington?" Rich asks him.

"Family." Zeus gives me a pointed look, and I squirm in my seat.

"Can you give us a minute?" I say to Zeus. "I just need to talk to Rich. It's work-related."

Zeus makes a snorting sound but doesn't say anything.

I scoot out of my seat and move away from our table with Rich following me.

I stop when we're out of earshot of anyone and turn to Rich.

Before I get the chance, he says quietly, "He's her dad," stating it, not asking.

"How?" I ask, flabbergasted.

"Well, I am a cop. It's my job to notice things like that. But, honestly, it's her eyes, Cam. She looks like you. But she has his eyes. They're a dead giveaway."

I trust Rich. He's not a gossip.

But I still say, "Please don't tell anyone. Gigi doesn't know yet."

"You can trust me, Cam. But how the hell does Gigi not know who her father is?"

"It's a long story."

"I have time."

"Not now. Another time," I tell him.

"We still on for Wednesday?"

I hesitate. "It's just difficult at the moment . . ."

"Okay," he says, running a hand through his hair. "I'm off the weekend after next. How about I take you out on Friday night?"

"We don't do that."

"I think we should. I like you, Cam."

"Are you asking because of Zeus?" I say and immediately regret it.

He frowns. "No. I've been asking you for a while now, Cam. Long before Zeus Kincaid showed up."

I glance down at my shoes. "Look . . . I like you, Rich. I do. But Gigi . . . she's going to find out soon who her father is. It's just not the right time for me to be starting anything up with anyone."

"We've been going for a while."

"We've been sleeping together," I say quietly. "A relationship is a whole other ball game."

He holds my eyes. "Okay, I get it. We'll put you and me on the burner until things calm down. But let me take you out next Friday, just as friends. You look like you could do with one right now."

I blow out a breath, giving in. "Okay. I'll check with

Aunt Elle and see if she's okay with watching Gigi. I'll text you and let you know for sure."

"Hastings," a voice calls from over by the counter.

"That's my order. So, I'll hear from you soon." He touches my hand with his.

"Yeah. I'll text you."

He walks away. I watch him for a second, and then I turn around to head back to our table. My eyes clash with Zeus's across the room.

He looks angry.

And, for a second, a feeling of guilt dips in my stomach. Like I've done something wrong.

But I haven't done anything wrong.

I just had a sensible conversation with a guy who, yes, I've slept with, but he's also my friend. And I need a friend right now.

Zeus was the one who screwed someone else, and then screwed me over.

He was the one who was just getting his flirt on with our waitress.

So, screw him. And, with that thought in mind, I tip my chin up and walk back over to our table.

Chapter Eleven

WHEN I SAT BACK down at our table, the atmosphere was a little strained between me and Zeus. But then the food arrived, and things got a little easier.

I hope, going forward, things will be easier and not be as strained, because we're going to have to be around each other, for Gigi's sake.

Zeus pulls the car up outside our house.

We get out. He helps Gigi from the car and then walks us up to our house.

I unlock the door and open it. "Thanks for today," I say to Zeus. "We had a nice time, didn't we, Gigi?"

"Yep. And *fank* you for Princess Twilight Sparkle." She hugs the toy to her chest.

"You are more than welcome." He smiles at her.

"Gigi, you go on inside. I'll be there in a minute. I just need to talk to Zeus."

"Can I watch TV?"

"Yes."

"Bye, *Zweus*." She waves at him.

"Bye, Gigi." He waves back. His voice sounds wistful.

I pull the door to a close once Gigi's inside. I hear the thud of her boots being abandoned in the hallway.

When I hear the TV come on in the living room, I start to speak, "I think today went well with you and Gigi." *Me and you, not so much.* "Gigi seems to really like you."

"I really like her." A smile touches his lips. "Not to be pushy, but when can I see her again?"

"She's at pre-K during the day tomorrow. But you can come for dinner tomorrow evening, if that works for you?"

"Yeah. That'd be great. What time should I come?"

"Four, if that isn't too early. Then, you can spend some time with her before dinner, which is at five thirty. She's usually bathed and in bed by six thirty, seven at the latest. If she doesn't get a full night's sleep, she's cranky. Gigi is not a morning person."

"Like you," he says.

His words poke at the sensitive part of me that remembers why he knows. All the mornings I woke up, wrapped in his arms.

And all the mornings since that I've woken up, alone and without him.

"So, four's okay?" I say.

"It's perfect."

"Okay, well . . ."

"Thanks for today, Cam," he says. "For letting me spend time with her. I really appreciate it."

"You don't have to thank me, Zeus. You're her . . ." I stop myself from saying *father*, as Gigi hears everything, and I don't want to risk it. "You have as much right as I do to spend time with her," I say in a quieter voice.

"Yeah." He exhales a sad sound, pushing his hand through his hair. "I know. It's just . . . I don't know." He shrugs, looking helpless. "It's surreal, you know."

I nod because I can only imagine what he's feeling.

"It'll get easier," I softly tell him.

"Yeah. But it won't get me back those four years."

There's a brief silence between us.

Then, I ask, "Have you spoken to Marcel?"

He shakes his head. "I'm waiting until I'm in a place in my head where I don't want to kill him."

"So, you'll be speaking to him in about ten years?" I say.

He laughs a sound from deep inside his chest. "Fuck, I've missed you, Dove," he says, surprising the hell out of me.

I have so many barbs on my tongue that I want to fire out, like, *Well, you wouldn't have had to miss me if you'd kept your dick in your pants*, but I bite them back and keep my mouth closed.

"I should get inside." I take a step toward the door. My hand is on the handle when his voice pulls me back.

"Why are you with him?"

I turn my face to him. "Who?"

"Deputy Dick."

"I'm not with him, Zeus. We're just friends."

"With benefits."

"I'm not discussing this with you."

"He's not good enough for you."

"And you were?"

"No." He steps closer to me. "I was never good

enough for you. I was just selfish back then, and I wanted you so fucking much."

Until you didn't.

I laugh, a bitter sound. "So, you cheating on me and dumping me was your way of being unselfish. Wow. I've heard some shit in my time, Zeus, but this . . ." I shake my head, disgusted.

"That's not what I meant."

"No? Then, what did you mean?"

Another step closer. So close that I have to tip my head back to look up into his face. He stares down into my eyes. The look in them is so intense, my insides start to tremble.

Then, he shakes his head and takes a step back. "You're not ready to hear it yet."

He starts to walk away from me.

My heart wants me to yell at him, *I'm not ready to hear what yet?*

But logic tells me to say, "I'm not interested in anything you have to say." And that's exactly what I do.

He stops at my words. His back turned to me. A few beats later, he looks over his shoulder at me. "I didn't give that waitress my number. If you were wondering."

"I wasn't," I say too quickly, giving myself away. I hate the relief I feel that he didn't give Megan his number.

A smile creeps onto his lips. "You always were a terrible liar, Dove. I'll see you tomorrow."

And yet again, he walks away from me, getting the last word in.

Chapter Twelve

IT'S BEEN ALMOST TWO weeks since Zeus showed up on my doorstep and discovered that he had a daughter. He's seen Gigi every single day. Even on Tuesday when she has a street dance class after pre-K. He asked if he could drop her off and pick her up. He also took her out alone on Sunday morning, to the movies to watch a reshowing of *Tangled*.

I did chuckle at the thought of Zeus Kincaid watching a Disney princess movie.

But it shows what he's willing to do to be with her. I can't fault him for his instant devotion to her. He's fallen hook, line, and sinker for our girl.

And she adores him, too.

Gigi still doesn't know that Zeus is her father. But I know we're getting close to that time.

Zeus hasn't once pushed the issue with me or asked when we're going to tell her the truth.

I guess I'm delaying it because I'm scared of her reaction. But also because it would make it real.

I need to be braver and tell her.

I'm thinking this weekend will be the best time. After her morning ballet class. Zeus has asked to take her. So, we can sit down together after that and tell her.

Zeus is here. He's in the living room with Gigi, playing Guess Who?—the *My Little Pony* version. He brought it with him for her.

It's the only other gift he's bought her since he got her Princess Twilight Sparkle that first day, so I don't mind too much. She takes that toy everywhere with her. I think it's partly because she always wanted one. But more so because Zeus bought it for her.

I'm in the kitchen, making dinner. We're having mac and cheese. Nothing too fancy. Zeus is staying for food, like he has every night. No Aunt Elle tonight, as she's at the station. She's not been home a lot at the moment. She's got some big case going on.

But she said she would watch Gigi tomorrow night for me, so I can go out for a drink with Rich.

I guess I could've asked Zeus to watch her for me, but it would've felt weird, asking him to babysit her while I'm out with Rich. Even though Rich is just a friend. I know Zeus has a problem with him. So, it's not worth the hassle.

It's hard, being around Zeus so much. Our relationship is strained, but we're cordial to each other. It's almost like we dance around each other. We exchange pleasantries. Yeses and noes. Pleases and thank yous. But not a real conversation.

If I'm being truthful, I still harbor a hell of a lot of anger and resentment for how he ended our relationship. But I have to bury that, for Gigi's sake. I have to pretend. That I never loved him. That he never broke my heart.

It's hard.

I still want answers from him that I never got.

The main questions being, *Why did he do it? Why did he cheat on me?*

If he had fallen out of love with me, then why not end things with me before dipping his dick in someone else?

I mean, I would have been heartbroken if he'd ended things with me because he didn't love me anymore. But to know that he had sex with another woman . . . it destroyed me.

And I've never really come to terms with those feelings. Because, a month later, I found out that I was pregnant with Gigi and was made to believe that he wanted nothing to do with her, so my anger for him turned to hate. I hated him for abandoning his child.

Now that I know that was never the case, my anger and resentment have swung back to what he did to me.

And, honestly, it's been feeling harder and harder to ignore it and pretend like I don't feel that way when I'm around him.

I pour the mac and cheese into a serving dish and grab the serving spoon. I carry them through to the dining room.

"Dinner's ready," I call as I pass through the hallway.

I put the mac and cheese down on the table, which I set with plates, silverware, a jug of water, and glasses before I started dinner. I head back to the kitchen to get the salad and garlic bread I prepared.

When I bring them to the table, Gigi and Zeus are already seated next to each other, waiting for me.

"I poured you a glass of water," Zeus tells me.

"Thanks," I say.

I put the salad and garlic bread on the table and take a seat across from them.

Zeus dishes up mac and cheese onto Gigi's plate for her. Then, he holds out a hand for mine. I pass my plate over and let him serve me. He hands me back my plate, and I put some salad on, too.

Zeus piles mac and cheese on his plate. I've had to double up on the food I usually make, as he has a huge appetite. He always has. But then he is a big guy, and he trains a lot.

We eat dinner, making small talk. Mainly, Gigi tells us about her day at pre-K. Zeus asks me about my day at work, so I tell him. And then I ask about his day.

It's all very domesticated. Too familiar.

I know it's because he's been spending every night eating with us. But I don't want Gigi getting too used to it, as it won't always be like this. Zeus won't always be here, in Port Washington, to eat dinner with her every night.

Maybe the sooner we tell Gigi that Zeus is her father, then we can figure out a routine for her to spend time with him. One that doesn't necessarily have to include the three of us being together all the time.

Mixed in with my anger toward him are also memories of the good times and reminders of why I fell in love with him all those years ago.

I'm like an assorted bag of emotions at the moment, fit to explode, and it's exhausting.

"Thanks for dinner. It was amazing, like always," Zeus says, leaning back in his seat.

"It was just mac and cheese." I put my fork down on my plate.

"You make the best mac and cheese, Mommy," Gigi says.

I smile at her. "Thanks, baby."

"So, you've cooked dinner and fed me every night," Zeus says. "And, as a thank-you, I want to take you out for dinner tomorrow night."

"Me?" I squeak, my pulse leaping.

A lazy grin spreads across his lips. "You and Gigi."

"Mommy can't go. She's going out with her *fwiend Wich*, the policeman, tomorrow night."

Crap.

The silence is deafening.

It's like a tumbleweed blowing through the dining room.

I force myself to look at Zeus. His face is clear of expression, his eyes blank.

I hate it when he does that. It means I can't get a read on what he's thinking.

"Well, I'm not going out until eight. But . . . I might be eating later."

Rich mentioned dinner after drinks.

"No problem," he says, his words a little clipped. "Is it okay if I still take Gigi to dinner?"

"*Pwease*, Mommy, can I go with *Zweus*?"

"Of course you can," I tell her.

"Yay!" Gigi claps her hands together.

"What time should I have her home?" he asks me. There's still an edge to his voice, which is starting to annoy me.

Why does he have such a problem with Rich?

You know why, a little voice whispers in my head.

Go away, Voice.

"Seven thirty at the latest," I tell him.

"And who's watching Gigi while you're out with Deputy Dick?"

"Who's Deputy Dick?" Gigi asks.

"No one. Zeus is just being silly." I glare at him.

He steadily stares back at me.

"Aunt Elle is watching her," I tell him, my voice harder than it was.

"Fine," he says roughly.

"Fine," I echo.

He pushes his chair out. My eyes follow him up.

"I gotta go, Gigi girl. But I'll be here at four thirty tomorrow to pick you up."

"Where we gonna eat, *Zweus*?"

"You can choose."

"Yay!" She claps her hands together again. "I's *fink* and tell you tomorrow."

His face softens, and he ruffles her hair with his hand. "Sounds like a plan." He casts a glance my way. "Thanks for dinner."

"No problem." I push to my feet. "I'll see you out."

"No need," he says. "I know where the door is. Bye, Gigi."

"Bye, *Zweus*."

I watch him leave and then sit back down in my seat, my stomach swirling with emotion.

It's clear that he's pissed because I'm going out with Rich.

And he has no right to be pissed.

The guy cheated on me, for God's sake!

Even still, I feel like I did something wrong when I didn't, and it's not fair of him to make me feel that way.

"Is *Zweus* mad, Mommy?"

My eyes swing to her. "No, of course he isn't."

"He looked angry."

"He'd never be angry with you."

"Not me, Mommy. You."

Crap.

I hate that my girl is so perceptive at times.

"I think he's just disappointed that I can't make dinner with you guys tomorrow night."

"You totally should come. *Zweus* and me are more fun than *Wich.*"

My brows furrow. "Do you not like Rich, Gigi girl?"

"He's okay. But I *wike Zweus* more."

My heart clenches painfully, and I realize that maybe Gigi has been picking up on more than I realized.

"You know that Rich is just Mommy's friend. Like Zeus is Mommy's friend."

"I know."

"And you know that it's good to have different friends."

"Yes, Mommy. But I *fink* people always *wike* one *fwiend* more than all the others. Like a best *fwiend.* And I *fink* you should be best *fwiends* with *Zweus.*"

I was. Once upon a long time ago.

Until he ruined it.

Unsure of how to respond to that, I get back to my feet. "Come on, Gigi girl. Let's clear these dinner plates away, and then you can watch some TV before bed."

Chapter Thirteen

I'M A COWARD.

After the frosty reception that I received from Zeus when he came to pick Gigi up to take her to dinner, I ensured I was already gone well before he was due to drop her back home.

I wasn't meeting Rich until eight, but I texted him and asked if we could meet earlier. Thankfully, he was able to; otherwise, I'd have been sitting in the bar alone for an hour before.

I'm sitting at a table that we snagged near the bar. Rich is up there, getting us drinks. I've asked for my usual—a Corona. It will be my one and only alcoholic drink for the evening. I'll be on soda after this. Rich offered to pick me up, but I prefer to be in my own car, so I can leave when I want. And not drinking more than one drink doesn't bother me.

As any mother knows, a hangover and a four-year-old do not go well together at all.

It's just nice to be out for a change and to also have a reason to get a little dressed up.

Not that I got overly dressed up. I'm wearing black skinny jeans, a sheer off-the-shoulder black top, and leopard-print ankle boots. My hair is down and straight, and I actually spent time doing my makeup. I went with red lips and smoky eyes. I look good, and for the first time since Zeus showed up, I feel good.

I get my cell out of my bag and check to make sure I haven't missed any calls or texts from Zeus or Aunt Elle about Gigi. Nothing. I place my phone on the table in front of me just in case.

When I lift my eyes, Rich is walking over with our beers. I watch as he comes toward me. He looks really good tonight in khakis and a button-down. It's not often that I get to see him in normal clothes. He's usually in his uniform—or naked—when I see him.

And . . . I'm not going there.

But I have noticed a difference in the way that I look at him tonight. Normally, when I see Rich, I get a zing of attraction in my chest—and other places. But, tonight . . . I don't feel it.

And it hasn't escaped my attention that my attraction to Rich has dwindled since Zeus showed up.

Damn you, Zeus Kincaid.

Rich reaches our table and puts down our drinks.

"Thanks," I say to him as he takes a seat across from me.

I pull my bottle toward me, take off the wedge of lime stuck to the lip of the bottle, and push it inside the neck with my finger.

"So, how've things been?" Rich asks me.

"You mean, with Zeus being back?"

Rich and I have texted a couple of times over the last few weeks but nothing in depth. I guess he was waiting until tonight to ask me.

"Hard. Stressful. Awkward. Strained." I give him a weak smile. "But Gigi's good. She's happy, and that's all that matters."

"Your happiness matters, too, Cam."

I lift my shoulder, not wanting to agree or disagree with him. Because Gigi will always come first. Even if that means my eternal misery.

Rich takes a drink of his beer before putting the bottle back down. "Do you want to talk about it? Zeus, I mean."

Sighing, I bring my bottle to my lips. "I don't really know what to say," I utter around the neck of my bottle before taking a sip.

"No pressure. Just know, I'm here to listen. And whatever you tell me will stay between us."

I smile gratefully at him. "It's just a really messed up situation." I start to pick at the label on my bottle. "I've known Zeus since I was fifteen. We were childhood sweethearts. I met him when I moved to Coney Island with Aunt Elle when she got a promotion there. We were together for four years. And then we weren't." I shrug. "Zeus was away a lot, training and doing fights. I was at Juilliard, studying ballet."

"I didn't know that. I knew you danced, but Juilliard? That's amazing, Cam."

"Yeah. I had a full scholarship. I was in my second year when Zeus and I broke up. He was in England at the time, training for a fight. He called me up one night. Told me that he'd slept with someone else."

Rich's face darkens at that. I don't know much about Rich's dating history. We've never talked about our pasts, but going by the look on his face, I'd say he's been cheated on, too.

"A month later, I found out I was pregnant with Gigi." And I go on to tell Rich the whole sordid story about Marcel and him lying to me and Zeus.

"Jesus," Rich murmurs. "That's . . . messed up."

"Yep."

"No wonder your head's all over the place. And, even though I'm hating on Zeus for cheating on you, I gotta feel for the guy as well. Not knowing he had a daughter for all those years? I can't imagine . . ." He trails off.

"Yeah, it's just all so awful. I feel sick for him. But, honestly, I do feel like I'm partly to blame for him missing out on Gigi's early years. Even though Marcel is a total bastard and lied to both of us, I feel like I should've done more to get in contact with Zeus."

"Cam, knowing you like I do, I'm sure you did everything you could."

I shrug, disagreeing, as I take another sip of my beer.

"Does Zeus blame you?"

"God, no." I shake my head for emphasis.

"Good," he growls. "Because he'd be an ass if he did."

I find myself feeling defensive of Zeus all of a sudden. "He's been great about it actually. He could have been a total ass, but he's been . . . great. He thinks it's on him for cutting me off in the first place. He blames himself for missing out on the first four years of Gigi's life. I feel sick when I think about it. I hate that she missed out on her father because of Marcel asshole

Duran. God, it all just feels like one big mess." I tear off the remainder of the bottle label and litter it onto the table.

"Things might be messy now, but it will get better," Rich assures me, touching my hand across the table.

"You think so?"

"I know so. You're a great mom, Cam. Gigi is an amazing little girl. And kids are resilient. It will all work out okay."

"I just . . . I don't know if I'm handling things the right way. Not telling Gigi from the start that Zeus is her dad."

"I don't think there's a set rule for a situation like this." He gives my hand a gentle squeeze, lacing a few fingers through mine. It doesn't feel sexual. It feels comforting. And I really need comfort right now. "I think you know your daughter best, and you're handling it the right way for her. What does Zeus think?"

"He's just following my lead. He hasn't been pressuring me at all to tell her."

"That's good, right?"

"Yeah." I sigh. "But it has also helped me delay the inevitable, you know."

He nods, picking up his beer.

"But I do think it's time though. It's been two weeks of them getting to know each other. Gigi thinks he's the best thing since sliced bread, which is great. She should. He's her dad. So, I'm hoping that she'll take it well when she finds out who he really is. I just think, if I let it go on longer, Gigi could resent me for not telling her sooner."

"That kid would never resent you. She loves you."

That makes me smile a little. “Yeah . . .” I muse. “I was thinking that I should tell her tomorrow. Well, that we—Zeus and I—should tell her after her ballet class. Not that I’ve had a chance to discuss it with Zeus yet to see what his thoughts are.”

“Well, you’ve got your chance now,” Rich says, eyes looking in the direction of the entrance. “Because he just walked in the bar.”

“Wha—” My head swivels on my neck. And there, filling out the doorway, looking as imposing and gorgeous as always, is Zeus.

And his eyes are narrowed and staring at me and Rich. Or more accurately, staring at Rich’s hand, which is still holding mine across the table.

Chapter Fourteen

I PUSH TO MY FEET, my hand pulling from Rich's, and I quickly make my way toward Zeus. My first thought being about Gigi.

"Is Gigi okay?" I ask as I approach him.

"She's fine."

I exhale in relief.

"She's at home with Elle," he adds. "I dropped her off about half an hour ago."

"Then, why are you here?" I blurt out.

His brows push together. "I came to catch the last part of the game." He nods in the direction of the TV hanging from the wall at the end of the bar, which is showing a football game. "I didn't know you'd be here, if that's what you're thinking."

"I wasn't." *I was.*

"If you say so."

"I do." I fold my arms over my chest. "Why in the world would I think that you came here for me?"

"I don't know, Dove. You tell me."

He's staring at me, and I'm starting to get flustered

and confused with the direction this conversation is going, which is the direction of . . . I don't have a clue.

"You really need to stop calling me that," I say, changing tactics.

"Dove? You never used to have a problem with me calling you it. You especially used to like me calling you it when I—"

"Don't . . ." I warn, knowing exactly where he's going with this.

Fire sparks in his eyes. "Don't what? Remind you of how you used to love me calling you Dove while I fucked you hard and deep."

I resist the shudder fighting to work its way through my body. My eyes scan the area to make sure no one heard what he just said.

"You're being inappropriate."

He laughs, but it's empty and hollow. "I haven't even started."

"What the hell is wrong with you?" I hiss.

His jaw works angrily. His eyes cutting through me. "Nothing, *Cam*." He emphasizes my name. "Not one single fucking thing is wrong with me." He tips his chin toward Rich. "Deputy Dick is waiting for you."

I turn my head to look over my shoulder at Rich. I give him a smile that's more forced than real.

When I look back to Zeus, he's no longer there.

My eyes zip across the space, seeking him out, to find him walking toward the bar.

The ass! He just walked away from me.

Well, if that doesn't just annoy the crap out of me.

I want to march over to him and say . . .

What, Cam? What do you want to say? And why

do you care so much that he just walked away from you?

I don't care. It's just . . . rude.

And I'm having an internal argument with myself.

Great.

I just need to talk to him about Gigi and telling her the truth tomorrow. We can't discuss it here. But he should know that we have to talk—sooner rather than later.

My eyes wander around the bar, and I can see people starting to take notice of him. It's only a matter of time before they start approaching him, and then I won't get a chance.

That's why I signal to Rich that I'll be back in a minute, and I walk over to where Zeus is now sitting on a stool at the bar, waiting to be served.

I tap his shoulder with my hand, and those blue eyes turn to look at me.

"You seen sense and ditched Deputy Dick?"

"I haven't ditched him. I just need to talk to you."

"About?"

"Not now. Tomorrow. You're still taking Gigi to ballet?" I check.

"Yes."

"Would you mind coming fifteen minutes earlier, so we can discuss something?"

"Sure."

"Great. Thanks."

An awkward silence starts to stretch between us. Zeus is staring at me, and I'm starting to feel jittery inside.

Walk away, Cam.

"Okay then"—I take a step back—"I'll see you tomorrow."

He gives me a brief nod before turning his attention to the bar. When the bartender approaches, Zeus gives his drink order—coffee.

He came to the bar to drink coffee?

No, he came to watch the game, stalker Cam.

I turn and skulk away, like a groupie who was just given the brush-off.

I reach our table and slip into my seat.

Rich, whose eyes were on his cell, looks up at me, putting his phone away in his pants pocket. "Everything okay?" he checks.

"Yeah, fine." I smile, way too big for it to be real. I pull my lips back together and try to relax my face. "I was just asking Zeus if he could come a little earlier tomorrow, so I can discuss the big talk with him."

"That's good." He nods.

"Yeah," I agree, picking up my half-drunk beer and taking a long swig.

Rich glances over his shoulder, looking toward the bar. "Hey, that's Zeus's brother, right?"

"Where?" I turn my head, half-expecting to see another Kincaid standing at the bar.

"On the TV. Playing for the Giants."

I lift my eyes to the television and see Ares's profile on-screen before he comes back into play. The sight of his face makes me smile. I always liked Ares.

Zeus told me that he hasn't told his siblings and his dad about Gigi yet. He wanted to spend time getting to know her first and then tell them after Gigi was told.

That will be tomorrow. Because I can't see Zeus disagreeing with telling her.

"He probably has box seats," Rich muses. "Wonder why he's in here, watching the game, and not actually there."

"He wanted to take Gigi"—*and me*—"out for dinner," I tell him, my eyes drifting to Zeus, unbidden.

He's talking to the bartender, and another guy at the bar has drifted over to talk to him.

"Ah. Right. That makes sense," Rich says. "So, did you hear about Larson?"

"No," I say, moving my eyes back to Rich.

"He's moving to Virginia," he tells me. "His mom lives there, and she's sick. He'd put in for a transfer on the DL, and it was approved today."

"That's good for him," I say. "Being closer to his mom."

"Yeah. It's going to be weird for me without him though. We went through the academy together . . ."

Voices lifting with excitement distract my attention from Rich, and I look back to the bar . . . to Zeus . . . where I now see that a group of women has swooped in on him, and they are falling all over themselves to talk to him.

"You're so big." One of them giggles as she wraps her hand around his biceps.

"That's what all the women say," Zeus replies.

Oh, for fuck's sake. I give a mental eye roll.

"You're so bad!" She laughs loudly.

Then, one of her friends pushes herself forward, wedging herself between Zeus and the bar, a pen held in her hand. "Will you sign my chest?" she asks him, sticking her enviably sized chest out, giggling and batting her lashes.

Really? Fucking really?

I grit my teeth, waiting for his response.

Then, I see a flash of that smile of his, and I'm hit with a tsunami of jealousy when Zeus takes the Sharpie from her hand and proceeds to sign her chest.

And I've seen enough.

"I'm not feeling great," I lie to Rich. "Sorry to bail early, but I'm gonna take off."

His eyes examine me, and then he looks over at Zeus before coming back to me. He knows I'm lying, and for a minute, I think he's going to call me out, but he says, "No problem. Let me walk you to your car."

"Sure." I smile.

We both stand. I grab my cell from the table and put it in my bag.

I can still hear the giggles of Zeus's groupies, but I don't look at him again.

When we get outside, the air is fresh, and it's just what I need to help clear my head.

We walk to my car in companionable silence. When I reach it, I get my keys out and unlock it.

I turn to Rich. "Thanks for tonight. For listening to me complain about my woes."

"Anytime." He smiles warmly. Then, he reaches out a hand and cups my cheek. "I like you, Cam."

"I like you, too." I smile. *I just wish I liked you more.*

He stares at me for a long moment, and I wonder if he's going to kiss me.

But he doesn't. He steps away and pulls open my car door for me.

I feel bad that I'm relieved.

I get in, put the key in the ignition, and pull on my belt.

"Drive safe," Rich says, holding the door. "I'll call you this week."

"Okay," I say.

He closes my door with a soft clunk, and I put it in gear and pull away, heading for home.

Five minutes later, I pull up onto my driveway behind Aunt Elle's car. The lights glowing from the living room tell me that Aunt Elle is still up.

But then, of course, she would be. It's embarrassing that I'm coming home early.

I suck at this going-out thing. But then I blame Zeus for turning up and ruining my night with his chest-signing antics.

On a sigh, I grab my bag and climb out of my car. I almost have a heart attack when I see Zeus standing at the end of my drive.

"Jesus Christ!" I say, clutching at my chest. "What the hell are you doing here? I thought you were still at the bar."

"I left when you did."

"Did you fly here?"

He laughs a deep sound that reverberates in my chest. "No. I just don't drive like a grandma."

"I don't drive like a grandma. I drive responsibly."

"Mmhmm." He chuckles that sound again.

"Why did you leave the bar? Did Busty's pen run out of ink?"

His lips lift into a sexy grin. "So, you did leave because you were jealous."

"I . . . what?" My mouth pops into an O. "No, I did not leave because I was jealous, Mr. Ego. There was nothing for me to be jealous over."

"If you say so."

"I do."

"Okay then." He turns and starts to walk back down the driveway.

I feel this harsh pull in my chest, and I'm speaking before I can stop myself, "What are you doing here, Zeus?"

He stops and turns around to face me. "Making sure you got home okay. I figured Deputy Dick wouldn't see you home unless he was getting something at the end of it."

"I went in my own car."

"He could have followed you home."

"How do you know he didn't?" I fire back.

He takes a step back and glances both ways down the empty street before giving me a pointed look. "Deputy Dick has a side job as the Invisible Man?"

"Fine," I snap. "He didn't see me home. But what does it matter to you?"

"You're the mother of my child. I care about your safety."

I let out a bitter laugh. "Just not for the last five years."

His face darkens, and he walks back to me, his long legs quickly eating the space between us. He stops inches away, and I suck in a breath.

"I fucked up, Cam." His voice is rough. "You think I don't know this? I know. Jesus, do I know. But I'm trying here." He scrubs a hand over his head. "I've made so many mistakes. But no more. I'm gonna do right by you and Gigi."

"I don't need you to do right by me. Only Gigi."

Zeus stares at me, and the look in his eyes makes me start to tremble.

"I don't think you understand, so I'm just going to make it plainly clear. I want you back."

"You . . . what?"

"I want you back."

He steps closer, and I instinctively step back, my heart rattling in my chest.

He frowns at my retreat but continues on, "I still love you, Cam. I never stopped."

"No. No fucking way. You don't get to come here and do this. We're over, Zeus. We were over a long time ago." *The moment you stuck your dick in someone else.* "The only thing between us now is that little girl sleeping upstairs."

He slowly shakes his head, his eyes holding mine. "We've never been over. I never moved on, and neither have you."

I grit my teeth, fury flooding in my veins. "I moved on a long time ago."

"No, Dove, you didn't. And you're lying to yourself if you think otherwise."

How dare he! How fucking dare he!

"You cheated on me!" I yell. "You slept with another woman behind my back, and then you told me over the phone when you were thousands of miles away! You broke my heart, Zeus! And I haven't seen or heard from you in five years. Now that you're back, you think you can just turn up here, saying these things, telling me you still love me? Well, you fucking can't!"

"I didn't cheat on you."

I stop. "What did you say?"

His eyes hold mine as he gently shakes his head. "I didn't cheat on you, Dove."

"But you said—"

"I lied."

Chapter Fifteen

Five Years Ago

AFTER A LONG DAY of classes, I climb into bed after brushing my teeth. I check my cell for messages before turning off the lamp, but there aren't any.

I was hoping to have a text from Zeus. I haven't heard from him in a few days. I sent some texts, but he hasn't replied to any of them. I know he's busy with training for this fight he's got coming up, and the time zone difference doesn't help. But it's not like him. He always makes contact with me every day when he's away.

I have this feeling . . . like dread. I've been trying to ignore it along with the voice in my head that keeps saying he's recently been pulling away from me.

But this is us.

Zeus and I are solid. We're the real deal.

I've loved the guy since I was fifteen years old.

It's just the long-distance thing. It's rough. But it'll get better. It has to.

I've just closed my eyes when my cell starts to ring.

My eyes flash open, and I grab my cell. My heart rate spikes at the sight of Zeus's name on the caller display. Even now, after all these years, he still has that effect on me. I hope it lasts for ever.

I connect the call. "Hey, handsome." A yawn escapes me, and I cover my mouth with my hand.

"Are you in bed?" Zeus's voice rumbles down the line.

"Yeah, but it's fine."

"I can call you tomorrow if that would be better."

"Zeus, I haven't talked to you in days. Now is better."

"Okay," he says.

"So, how's training going?" I ask.

"Good. Look, Cam . . ."

He called me Cam. He rarely calls me Cam. Only when he's pissed at me or he has something to tell me that I'm not going to like.

"Are you gonna be in England for longer than expected?"

"No, it's not that."

"Then, what?"

His silence down the line worries my insides.

"Zeus, what's going on?" I swallow, nervously.

He clears his throat. "I've been thinking . . . and . . . well . . . I think we should spend some time apart."

"Spend time apart?" I echo.

"Yes."

I start to worry my bottom lip with my teeth. "I don't understand."

"Space, Cam," he snaps. "I need space."

My stomach bottoms out, and panic clutches at my throat. "But I hardly ever see you."

"Exactly. I just think it would be better for us if we took a break."

A break.

I've seen *Friends*. "The One Where Ross and Rachel Take a Break." Ross screwed the copy machine girl in that episode.

I don't want to take a break.

And the fact that he does is scaring the shit out of me.

"Zeus, are you . . ." I swallow what feels like a brick down my throat. "Are you breaking up with me?"

The silence that follows is agony.

"Yes."

And the agony turns into a pain, the likes of which I've never known. I feel like my heart is being ripped in two.

Tears flood my eyes. I press the phone harder against my ear, needing to feel something, anything, but this agony he's inflicting on me.

"Zeus, please . . . don't do this. I know the long-distance thing has been hard—"

"We've seen each other three times in the last six months."

"We saw each other last week!" I sob.

"For one night. That's not a relationship."

"Jesus, Zeus. Don't do this. Please. I love you." My pride has gone out the window.

This is Zeus. I'd do anything to keep him with me. He's the love of my life. The only guy I've ever been with. A life without him just doesn't seem feasible. In my mind, I've shaped my whole future around him.

Every single memory I planned on making has him in it, and now, he's telling me that he doesn't want to be a part of that anymore.

He doesn't want me anymore.

I can't breathe. I feel like there's a hand around my throat, choking me. His hand.

"Please, Zeus. We can make it work. I'll fly out to England on the next flight. I've got some money on my credit card. We can talk and—"

"I don't want you to come."

It's like he's stuck a blade in my gut.

"You just want to throw the last four years away like they don't matter?" I whisper, brushing tears from my cheeks.

Silence.

The only thing I can hear is his breathing down the phone.

"I'm not in love with you anymore, Cam. I'm sorry."

The blade pulls out of my gut and sinks in my heart.

Don't be sorry, I want to scream. *Just fucking love me.*

I start to choke on my tears. "You don't mean that. We've just spent so much time apart that you've forgotten how good we are together. I'm gonna leave Juilliard and come to you—"

"No," he says firmly.

I ignore him. I can't hear him. I don't want to hear him.

"We can spend some time together, and we'll be okay. You'll see me and remember that you love me and—"

"I slept with someone else."

If I thought hearing the other things hurt me, then I had no clue what real pain was.

I've never felt anything like what I'm feeling now. It's

like my heart has turned into glass, and he just punched his fist through my chest, shattering it into a million pieces.

I go still. Numb. The tears that fall down my cheeks are the only thing I can feel.

"Cam . . ."

I disconnect the call and throw my cell at the wall. I hear it shatter, like my heart just did.

I stare into the darkness as fresh tears run down my face, dripping onto my nightshirt.

Zeus's shirt. One of his old T-shirts that I stole to wear to bed.

He had sex with another woman.

He cheated on me.

Zeus. My Zeus.

But he's not mine anymore.

A cry of raw agony rips from my lungs.

I pull his shirt from my body and hurl it across the room, needing anything of his far away from me.

I fall to the bed, curl up into a ball, and cry until there are no more tears left inside me.

A week later, I see Zeus pictured in the papers with another woman.

A month after that, I discover that I'm pregnant with his baby.

Chapter Sixteen

"YOU DID WHAT?" I gasp, stepping back from him.

Zeus at least has the decency to look guilty. "I lied. I never cheated on you."

I feel winded. I know I should feel relieved, but I don't. Everything I've believed for the last five years—that Zeus cheated on me, that he abandoned Gigi—none of it is true. And I don't know how to feel right now.

"W-why did you do that?"

He sighs and drives a hand through his hair. "Because I knew it was the only way that you'd let me go."

Jesus.

Tears burn the back of my throat. "You wanted to get rid of me so badly that you lied and told me you'd slept with another woman when you hadn't?" My hands cover my chest, clutching at the pain there.

"I didn't want to get rid of you, Cam. I thought I was doing the right thing at the time."

"By lying to me?"

"It wasn't like I'd planned on it. You started talking about leaving Juilliard again, and I panicked."

"Again? That was the first time I even mentioned leaving Juilliard!"

He slowly shakes his head, holding my eyes. "You'd been hinting at it for months."

Had I?

I loved being at Juilliard, but I loved Zeus more. Constantly being away from him was getting harder and harder, overshadowing my feelings toward everything else.

"It was hard, being away from you all the time," I tell him my thoughts. "But I was willing to stick it out until we could get back to the way things were. You were the one who walked away."

"That's just it. Things were never going to go back to the way they were. Our lives had changed, and we were being pulled in two separate directions. I couldn't let you give up Juilliard for me. Not when I couldn't give you what you deserved—all of me. What with the constant training, fights, and strict regimes I was under. It just felt impossible. And Marcel was always on my back about you. Telling me that you were a distraction. Getting in my head, saying that, if I wanted to achieve anything, I needed one sole focus—boxing. After every single time I spoke to you on the phone, Marcel would say my head wasn't in it. That I was distracted. And he was right. You remember how I got this?" He touches the scar on his eyebrow.

"Of course I remember." My words are soft.

Zeus came to visit me on some downtime he had after his first big fight post-Olympics. We were out at a club. A guy was hitting on me. Zeus saw red. There was an argument. A fight broke out. The guy grabbed a beer bottle and hit Zeus with it. I'd never seen so much blood in all my life, and I'd been watching his fights since I was fifteen.

The doctor said he was lucky he didn't lose his eye.

"Marcel wanted you gone then. That wasn't your fault. I knew that. But he said it would never have happened if I hadn't been with you. He said I was fucking up my career over you. That I had a chance to change my family's life, but if I kept on as I was, that would never happen. I was going to screw everything up. He got in my head, and I let him.

"And I was just so fucking worried about you all the goddamn time because you were unhappy with our situation, and there was nothing I could do to fix it or change things. I could've stopped boxing and come home, but then what would I have done? Work in some shitty factory for the rest of my life? I needed money to support Ares, the twins, and my dad. I was trapped, Cam. And something had to give."

"And that something was me."

I wrap my arms around myself.

"I thought you'd be better off without me," he says quietly. "I thought, if I sacrificed my own happiness by letting you go, that I would be doing the right thing for my family. You'd get over me. You'd move on and have this amazing career as a dancer.

"But then, when I saw you in the club that night, dancing on that fucking podium, with that asshole trying to feel you up . . ." He breathes out heavily. "You were supposed to be onstage at the New York City

Ballet, for fuck's sake. Right there and then, I knew I'd screwed up.

"But, when I came here and found out about Gigi . . . Jesus." He grabs the back of his neck, tipping his head back to the dark sky. "I'd given you up, and it was all for nothing. And, even worse, I'd missed out on four years of my daughter's life."

I don't know what to say, so I say nothing. My mind is racing with everything he just told me.

"Cam . . ." he says my name softly, pulling my eyes to his.

What I see there halts all thought. He moves closer to me, leaving mere inches between us. I can feel the heat from his body. My pulse starts to race.

"Letting you go was the hardest thing I've ever had to do." His voice is rough. "Harder than watching my mother's body being lowered into that grave. I loved you so much, Dove. I still do. I've never stopped loving you. And I've spent the last five years missing you."

His words touch all the bruised parts inside me, like a soothing balm. But I can't let him get close. It's too much.

All of it.

Panic grips my chest like a vise.

And, when he reaches a hand out to touch me, I move back, wrapping my arms around my chest.

"It's too late, Zeus. We're different people now. *I'm* different."

He shakes his head. "You're still the same. You're still my little Dove."

"I . . . you're not being fair. You can't say these things to me. And how am I supposed to believe a word you say? You admit that you lied to me about something so hurtful as cheating on me."

"It's the only time I've ever lied to you."

"I honestly don't know what to believe anymore. All you seem to do is throw bombs at me and then walk away, leaving me to clean up the mess."

"Believe that I love you. I want you. And I'm not going anywhere."

"Until you disappear to train for weeks on end for the Dimitrov fight."

He erases the space I just put between us, and I find myself backed up to the front of the porch.

"I'm not leaving you or Gigi, Dove. I'm here to stay. Wherever my girls are, I'll be. Port Washington is my home now. That's why I left the hotel, and I'm renting an apartment."

My heart lurches and reaches for him. He never once mentioned that he was looking for a place to rent. I just assumed he'd stay in the hotel until he had to start training for the Dimitrov fight.

He's saying all the right things. Doing all the right things. Everything I wanted from him years ago. But, now . . . it's too late.

I can't risk my heart on Zeus again. I have Gigi to think of now.

I steel myself, putting the walls back up, and slip out from between him and the porch.

His body follows me around.

"That's really great. For Gigi's sake. But don't do anything with me in mind, Zeus. Because we're not happening. I don't trust you anymore."

"I'll earn it back," he counters.

I shake my head. "It's too late."

"No, it's not."

"Don't fool yourself into believing that."

"I'm not giving up on you . . . on us."

"Well then, you'll be wasting your time. Put your focus on our daughter, Zeus. And forget about me."

"I haven't been able to forget about you in the last five years, so I can't see it ever happening."

I walk away from him, heading for the porch, so done with this conversation. "Go home, Zeus."

I hear him sigh behind me.

"Before I do . . . in the bar, you said you wanted to talk to me in the morning. What's it about?"

I turn to face him, standing on the porch steps. "I think we should tell Gigi who you really are. Tomorrow, after her ballet class."

A multitude of emotions crosses over his face. All of them good. "You're sure?" he checks.

I nod.

"Thank you."

"Don't thank me yet. Let's see how tomorrow goes first." I walk to the door, rubbing my hands over my arms, warding off the chills I feel at the thought of the day to come and the night I've just had. The night I'm still having.

My thoughts have somewhat calmed, and I pause before opening the front door to ask him something.

Something that I need the answer to.

When I turn, I find him still standing on the driveway, eyes watching me.

"Zeus . . ." My voice suddenly sounds amplified in the silence. "If you hadn't seen me in the club that night, would . . . you have ever come back for me?" I have to know this. It matters a lot.

His eyes lower to the ground. He pushes his hands into his pockets, the toe of his boot kicking at the gravel. "I don't know." His words are quiet. "I wanted to come back. God, I wanted to. I just . . ." He sighs and lifts his head, finally meeting my eyes. "I just didn't know how to."

Even though I anticipated this, hearing it still hurts like a mother.

A sound of expected disappointment leaves me. "And that's the reason I'll never believe a single thing you tell me, Zeus. Because, when you love someone—*really* love them—you fight for them. You fight hard and dirty, no matter the cost to yourself. And not *once* have you ever fought for me."

And, with those parting words, I open the door and step inside, firmly shutting it behind me.

Chapter Seventeen

I'M PACING THE FLOOR, chewing on my thumbnail, as I anxiously wait for Zeus to return from ballet class with Gigi. While she's been gone, I've kept myself busy with cleaning the kitchen. Gigi's class ended ten minutes ago, so she'll be home any minute.

When Zeus came to pick her up an hour ago to drive her there, we barely spoke a word.

He just asked me if we were still going ahead with telling her after class. And I said yes.

That was the extent of our conversation.

We didn't talk about last night.

I can't talk about last night. Or think about any of the things he said last night. Because today is too important for anything else to come in the way of it.

I just pray to God that Gigi is okay with what we're about to tell her.

I hear the door open and the sound of Gigi chattering away with Zeus.

Then, she calls for me, "Mommy!"

This is it. Time to woman up and tell my girl the truth.

"Living room," I say.

She comes running into the room, a whirl of pink and frills, and launches herself into my arms. "Guess what!" She presses her tiny hands to my cheeks.

"What?" I say.

Zeus walks into the room, and my eyes briefly go to him. He's wearing a smile, but I can see the worried look in his eyes.

I try to give him a reassuring smile, but I don't think it works.

"You has to guess, Mommy. Or it's no fun."

"Okay, I'll guess. But you have to give me a clue."

Her little nose screws up, and then she grins. "Okay. Do you see *anyfing* different 'bout me?" She removes her hands from my face and spreads her arms out wide.

I spotted the badge pinned to her leotard straightaway, but I play dumb.

I tip my head back and pretend to examine her face. "Hmm . . . well, it's not your face because it looks the same."

"*Cwourse* it does, Mommy. Don't be silly. I can't change my face."

I don't even bother to tell her about the wonders of plastic surgery.

"Good. Because I love your pretty face just the way it is."

I kiss the tip of her nose, and she giggles.

"Come on, Mommy, guess! *Zweus* guessed way *qwicker* than you!"

"Oh." I lift a playful brow, giving Zeus a teasing look. "Is that so? Well, we can't have that." I scan my eyes over her and then say, "You wouldn't be Ballerina of the Week by any chance, would you?"

"You guessed *wight*! I'm the best dancer this week. Miss Hannah said my *fwirst* position was perfect. And I said that's because I been *pwacticing* at home. And she said that I'm going to make a *gweat* ballerina. And I said just *wike* my mommy."

The wave of love I feel for her, almost takes my breath away. I press my lips to her warm cheek and breathe in her scent. "I'm really proud of you, Gigi girl." I hug her to me before putting her to her feet. "So, Zeus and I need to talk to you about something, if that's okay."

She looks up at me. "Okay, Mommy."

I take her hand and lead her over to the sofa. She sits down on the sofa, and I sit beside her. Zeus sits on her other side.

"So, Gigi . . . there's something that Zeus and I need to tell you."

"Are you and *Zweus* getting *mwarried*?"

"What? No!" I splutter.

My eyes flash to Zeus. He doesn't look upset by that. If anything, he's smiling.

"Why would you think that, baby?"

"Because Tommy Preston told me that his mommy gots a new friend *wike* we gots *Zweus*, and nows, they *mwarried*."

"No, Gigi girl. Zeus and I aren't getting married." I gently shake my head.

"Okay. But I wouldn't mind if you dids. I *wike* Zeus a *wot*."

She gives me a toothy grin, and I can't help but smile at her.

I lift my eyes to Zeus, and the sheer level of emotion on his face almost breaks me.

I swallow down composing myself, before attempting speech again.

"So . . . Gigi girl, you know how Tommy's mom got married to her friend, and that meant he got a new daddy?"

"Tommy has two daddies. I don't has a daddy," she tells Zeus. There's no hurt in her voice. Just a matter of fact. But it's still like a blade in the heart.

Zeus clears his throat. "Well, what would you say if I told you that I was your daddy?" His voice is like gravel.

Gigi's just staring at him. And my heart is practically beating out of my chest.

"So, you wants to be my daddy?"

"Well, Gigi, I am your daddy."

She turns her eyes to me, looking confused.

"Do you understand what we're telling you, baby?"

"*Zweus* is my daddy."

"Yes, Gigi girl, Zeus is your daddy." I reach out and take hold of her hand.

She looks back to Zeus, who looks absolutely terrified. "I's known my mommy forever," she says to him. "Why hasn't I's known you forever if you's my daddy?"

Jesus. Grief clamps down on my heart, and the pain in Zeus's eyes nearly rips me wide open.

He takes her other hand, engulfing it with his. "It's difficult to explain, Gigi." His voice is raw with anguish.

"But I want you to know that I didn't want to *not* know you. I didn't know . . . that you . . . were . . ." He's faltering, and I don't know if I should step in and help or not. "Gigi, if I had known about you, then I promise that I would have known you forever, just like your mom has."

"Okay."

"Okay?" he echoes.

She smiles at him, pulling her hand from mine, and pats his hand that's holding hers. "S'okay, *Zweus*."

Well . . . hell.

I guess, sometimes, it's just that easy with kids.

"Do I has to call you Daddy now instead of *Zweus*?"

He clears his throat. "Not if you don't want to. It is up to you—what you choose to call me."

She stares at his face for a long moment, head tilted, pondering it. "I *fink* I'll call you Daddy. All my *fwiends* at school have a daddy, and I always wanted one. So, now, I can tell *evewyone* that I has a daddy, too."

Emotions crash into me like a punch to the stomach, watering my eyes and clogging my throat. I fight back my feelings and paste on a smile as Gigi turns to me.

"Can I's have a snack now?" she asks.

I briefly close my eyes, loving my girl so much in this moment. "Sure you can. Go get changed out of your ballet clothes, and I'll have your snack ready for you when you come down."

"Okay, Mommy." She hops off the sofa and then pauses in the open doorway. "Can I's have potato chips?"

"Yes."

"And *chocowate*?"

I'd give her the moon right now if she asked. Still, I find myself grinning. "Okay, Gigi girl. But that's all."

I swear, kids can smell weakness in their parents and know exactly when to ask for what they want.

"You da best, Mommy!" she sings. "And you, too, *Zweus*—I mean, Daddy." She slaps her hand to her forehead, being silly, and then she's gone, thundering up the stairs.

"Jesus H Christ," Zeus breathes, his hands going to his face, covering it and then pushing up into his hair.

"Yeah," I exhale. "That went . . . better than I expected."

"She's amazing," he says, sounding awestruck.

"She is."

"And, when she called me Daddy . . . God, Cam . . ." His eyes lift to mine, and they're glittering. "I've never felt anything like that before."

"I know," I say.

I touch his hand with mine on instinct.

And, just like that, the air charges and sparks with memories of heated touches and long kisses.

I stand abruptly, running a hand over my hair, smoothing it down. "I should go make our girl's snack, because she'll be down in a minute."

And I walk out of the room to the feel of Zeus's eyes on my back.

Chapter Eighteen

IT'S BEEN A FEW weeks now since we told Gigi that Zeus was her father, and she's adapted to the news without a hitch. She's transitioned to him being her dad so well, it worries me that she hasn't acted out more.

Or maybe that's just me being an overprotective parent.

Zeus has been spending more time with just Gigi. Taking her out and doing things together. I think it's important because, if it's always the three of us doing stuff together, then Gigi could get the wrong impression. It showed that was already happening when we sat her down to talk to her, and she thought I was going to tell her that Zeus and I were getting married.

It makes it easier that Zeus has a place here now, as he can take her there as well, so we're not here all the time.

Although, today, we're all here together.

But there's a good reason for that.

Zeus's family is coming to meet Gigi. Well, Ares, Lo, and Missy are. He told me that he's not letting her meet his dad until he's sobered up. And, from what he last told me about Brett's failed attempts at rehab, I don't think Gigi will be meeting him anytime soon, but I wholeheartedly agree with Zeus's decision.

I don't want an addict brought into Gigi's life. Even though I don't remember my mother, I know how she was. Addicts care about only one thing—their addiction—and nothing else.

So, the Kincaid clan is coming here today to meet Gigi. Apparently, they've been hassling Zeus to come and meet Gigi after he told them about her. He's been holding them off for as long as he could, but he finally caved under pressure.

Gigi was really excited to find out that she had two uncles and an auntie. After having just me and Aunt Elle for so long, it must be amazing for her to have all these new people in her life.

Missy and Lo have been home from college for the weekend to meet Gigi. They're staying with Ares in New York because his place is bigger than Zeus's.

Zeus is renting a two-bedroom apartment on Main Street that overlooks the water.

It's nice but basic. But that's Zeus. He's never been one to go for the flash.

The only reason he's ever fought is to earn money to care for his siblings.

How did I ever think that he could've walked away from Gigi?

But then, I wasn't exactly in the best place at the time, and I believed that he'd slept with another woman, and I was dealing with finding out he wasn't the man I'd thought he was. So it was easy to be tricked into believing that he wanted nothing to do with his unborn child.

"All ready?" Aunt Elle wanders into the kitchen where I'm just finishing up prepping the food for the Kincaids.

I thought it would be nice to make it like a little party for Gigi. Meet-the-other-half-of-your-family-for-the-first-time kind of thing. So, I've made sandwiches and finger food along with some cupcakes. I just want it to be nice for everyone.

"Yeah, all ready." I smile a little too brightly for it to be real.

"It's gonna be all right, Cam."

"You've been saying that a lot recently."

"Yeah, and I've been right every time."

I'm feeling really nervous about seeing them after all this time. I'm worried that they blame me for Zeus not knowing about Gigi.

Aunt Elle is staying for moral support—or, in her words, she's here in case anyone upsets me, so she can kick their ass.

Zeus assures me that they don't blame me, just like he doesn't.

I didn't openly volunteer my concerns to him. He just knew.

And that's because he knows me. He knows my tells when I'm worried or nervous.

And, last night, after putting Gigi to bed—he's been staying to tuck her in and read her a story, and then he leaves and goes back to his apartment—I was in the kitchen, making the cupcakes for today, feeling stressed, and he came in and asked me what was worrying me.

I said, "Nothing."

He said, "Bullshit."

Then, he told me what I was worrying about and then set about reassuring me.

Sometimes, I hate that he knows me so well.

It makes everything so much harder.

I've been trying to process what he told me. That he never cheated on me. That he's still in love with me.

Truthfully, I don't know what to do with it.

He hasn't said any more about it since that night, and I'm glad for that because it's not something I want to face right now.

I love Zeus. I always have. He's Gigi's father. I'm always going to feel something for him. And, of course, I'm attracted to him. It's Zeus, for God's sake. The man is the walking epitome of sex.

But I don't trust him.

I trust him one hundred percent with Gigi. I know he'd protect her with his life.

I don't trust him with my feelings.

I've been hurt by Zeus Kincaid once before. I'm not looking for a repeat performance.

And, honestly, I'm starting to wonder if my parting words that night resonated with him. That he doesn't love me the way he thinks because he's never fought to be with me.

And, if that is the case . . . then, I don't know how I feel about that either.

God, aren't I just a mixed bag of emotions right now?

And it's all because of that man who's currently sitting in my living room.

But today is about Gigi. She's my main priority. My only priority.

"Gigi still in the living room with Zeus?" I ask Aunt Elle, who's started helping me wrap the plates of sandwiches.

But, before she can answer, the doorbell rings. There's an excited squeal from the living room and then the sound of Gigi and Zeus heading toward the front door.

"Guess that's them." I smooth my hands down my dress. I thought I'd make an effort, so I put on my nicest day dress—a white floral maxi.

"Showtime, kid." Aunt Elle winks at me and grins.

I head out of the kitchen and into the hallway. The front door is open, Gigi standing there with Zeus, and on our porch stand Ares, Lo, and Missy. They're all smiling down at my girl.

It's been five years since I've seen them.

Ares looks the same, just older. He's always been big, like Zeus. They're both similar but different, too. They have the same eyes. All of them have those striking blue eyes, which must have come from their mom, as Brett's eyes aren't like that. But where Zeus's hair has always been short, Ares keeps his long. It's tied back into one of those man buns, and he's wearing a lot of scruff on his face.

Lo was sixteen the last time I saw him. He was tall then, but now, he's twenty-one and standing as tall as Zeus, just not as muscular. More athletic-looking.

And Missy is stunning. She was a pretty girl when she was a kid, but she's grown into a beautiful young woman. Tall, like her brothers, she's around my height, and looking at her now, I can see some of Gigi in her, or vice versa.

Zeus picks Gigi up, so she's at eye-level with them. And I hang back with Aunt Elle at a safe distance, watching them.

"Gigi, this is your uncle Ares," Zeus indicates.

"Hey, Gigi." Ares smiles at her. "It's good to finally meet you. I've heard a lot about you from your daddy."

"Daddy told me you play *fwootball*," she says.

"You like football?" he asks her.

"S'okay, I guess. But I *wikes* to dance."

"Yeah, and I've heard you're really good at it."

She beams at him. "I *pwactise* all the time."

"Gigi, this is your uncle Lo and your aunt Missy."

"Hey, Gigi," they say at the same time.

"Do you *pway* football, too?" she asks Lo.

He chuckles and shakes his head. "No, I leave the sports to your dad and Uncle Ares."

"Look how beautiful she is, Z." Missy steps closer to Gigi. "She has mom's eyes. God, I'm so happy to meet you, Gigi. Would it be okay if I hugged you?"

Gigi looks to Zeus for consent, and he nods at her.

Missy reaches out and hugs her while Gigi's legs stay attached to Zeus's hips.

Missy leans back, taking Gigi's face in her hands. "I'm gonna spoil you so bad." Missy grins at her.

I decide, thanks to the gentle dig in my ribs from Aunt Elle, that it's time for me to say my hellos and invite them in, as they're all still standing outside on the porch.

"Hey, guys." I walk toward them, smiling.

The greeting I get isn't one I was expecting.

"Cam!" Missy squeals and then runs through the

doorway at me, throwing her arms around my neck, almost knocking me off my feet.

"Hey." I chuckle, a little winded, hugging her back.

She leans back, grinning into my face. "I can't believe how long it's been! And you look even more gorgeous than ever, ya biatch—oops! Shit!" She covers her mouth, giggling. "Gotta learn to watch my mouth," she says between her fingers.

"Yeah, you do," Zeus grunts from behind.

"It's good to see you, Missy."

"You, too." She smiles at me.

Lo comes over and kisses me on the cheek. "Thanks for inviting us, Cam."

"Oh, no problem at all."

They go over to say hello to my aunt Elle as Ares meanders over to me.

"Cam."

"Hey, Ares." I smile, not sure how to greet him.

He's the one I've been most worried about hating me, as he's always been closest to Zeus. I mean, they're all close. But, with Lo and Missy being twins, they are naturally close. Zeus and Ares have always looked out for one another. They're brothers in the truest sense of the word.

Then, he steps forward, puts his huge arms out, and hugs me. "Missed you," he says.

I feel a wave of emotion.

Zeus was the love of my life. But Ares was my friend. We went to high school together, and after Zeus left to get a job and box full-time, Ares was the one to watch out for me at school. When Zeus and I broke up, I didn't just lose him; I lost my friend, too.

Freeing his arms from around me, he steps back and looks me in the eyes. "You're not getting rid of us now, you know. We're here to stay."

He grins, and I laugh softly.

"Glad to hear it."

Zeus comes over with Gigi still in his arms.

"Mommy, can we eat now?"

"Sure, Gigi girl." I smile at her. "Why don't you take our guests into the living room, and I'll bring the food through?"

"I'll give you a hand," Zeus says.

"And I'll grab the drinks," Aunt Elle announces.

Chapter Nineteen

"THANKS AGAIN FOR INVITING us," Missy says to me as we all reach the door.

They're leaving, as Ares has to be up early for practice. It's well past Gigi's bedtime, and she's starting to tire.

"You're welcome anytime," I tell her.

"You're gonna regret saying that." She chuckles, and I laugh, opening the door for them.

But I can't imagine ever regretting it. Today has been really great. I was totally worried for no reason.

We all got along great. It was like old times. At one point, we were even all out back, playing a game of football, as Gigi wanted Ares to show her how to play. Even Aunt Elle joined in.

It was fun.

But, now, Gigi's saying she wants to play football.

Not sure how that will go over with Miss Hannah, her ballet teacher, but if my girl wants to learn to play football, then she can.

But, mainly, they doted on Gigi. And she loved the attention.

I have a feeling that my girl has each and every one of the Kincaids wrapped around her little finger.

Lo and Ares say their byes to Gigi, and I receive a kiss on the cheek from each of them before they step outside with Zeus.

Aunt Elle's not here. She said her good-byes earlier. She had gotten a call about an hour ago and had to head into the station.

Missy drops to one knee in front of Gigi. "So, I'll see you real soon, Gigi. And your mom has my number now, so we can FaceTime whenever you want."

"I'll set it up on her iPad, so she can call you," I tell Missy. "But you do realize that you'll probably get calls at six in the morning."

"No problem at all. I'm usually up early."

"You mean, up late and coming home at six," Lo grunts from outside the door.

She rolls her eyes and says, "I have no idea what you mean, little brother."

Missy is older by five minutes, and she doesn't let Lo forget it.

She focuses her attention back on Gigi. "Can I have a hug from my gorgeous niece before I go?"

I love how she always asks Gigi for her permission before hugging her. I hate it when relatives force kids to hug and kiss them.

"Of *cwourse* you can, Aunt Missy!" Gigi giggles and launches herself at Missy, nearly knocking her over.

"Steady, Gigi," I say.

"She's fine." Missy chuckles. "Best tackle hug I've ever received. We'll make a football player out of you yet."

She gently tweaks Gigi's nose and then gets to her

feet. She comes over to me and wraps her arms around me. "Thank you, Cam," she says quietly. The emotion I hear in her voice puts a lump in my throat. "This is the happiest I've seen Zeus in a long time." She pulls back and looks me in the eyes. "He . . . told me that you're seeing someone. A cop?"

My eyes seek out Gigi, and I see she's outside with the men.

Missy drops her voice even lower, recognizing my concern. "I just wanted to say that I hope you're happy. You deserve to be."

I swallow back my emotion. "I'm not . . . I mean, I am happy. But that's not because of Rich. And I don't know exactly what Zeus told you, but the thing with Rich . . . it's not serious. Honestly, I don't even know if I'm seeing him anymore. Things are . . . complicated at the moment."

My eyes flicker to Zeus without permission. He's laughing at something Ares just said. His smiling eyes meet mine, and something tugs painfully in my chest.

"He's never gotten over you," Missy softly tells me, pulling my eyes back to hers. "And something tells me that you've never gotten over him either."

I press my lips together, not wanting to say anything because I'm not sure what to say.

"God, sorry." She screws up her face. "I'm overstepping, like usual. Just tell me to mind my own business."

"You're fine. It's just . . ."

"Complicated," she finishes for me.

"Yeah." I sigh.

"Life would be a hell of a lot simpler if things weren't though, right?"

I nod my agreement.

She presses a kiss to my cheek. "Thanks again, Cam. And, next time, I promise to keep my opinions to myself."

I smile at her before she turns away.

"Right, come on, boys." She claps her hands together. "Let's leave Cam in peace."

"What? You were the one holding us up by chatting with her," Lo grumbles.

She passes him, going down the porch steps. "I wasn't chatting. I was talking."

"Isn't that the same thing?"

"No."

"I think, if you check the dictionary, you'll find it is."

"Shut up, Lo."

"Jesus, I'm gonna have to listen to you two bitching all the way home?" Ares complains as they start to walk down the driveway toward Ares's car.

"So long as Lo doesn't talk, we should be fine," I hear Missy say.

I laugh.

Zeus picks up Gigi and comes over to stand beside me. She rests her head on his shoulder, her eyes drooping.

"Bedtime," I say to her.

She must be tired because she doesn't even complain.

"You want me to put her down?" Zeus asks.

"That'd be great," I tell him. "I'll get the house cleaned up."

I do kind of miss putting Gigi to bed, but I've had four years of doing it, so I figure it's only right to let Zeus do it for now.

"If you wait, I'll help you when I come down."

"It's fine." I wave him off. I give Gigi a good-night kiss. "Night, baby."

"Night, Mommy," she mumbles, sounding exhausted.

"Maybe skip brushing her teeth tonight," I tell Zeus, "and just put her straight to bed."

"Got it," he says.

I watch him carry her upstairs, emotion swelling inside me at the sight of them together like that.

I swear, every time I see Zeus carrying her, my ovaries do a shimmy, and I can't help but think, *What if . . .*

Shaking my head clear of those thoughts, I head into the kitchen and start on the cleanup.

I've just finished filling the dishwasher up when Zeus comes in.

"She asleep?" I ask.

"The second her head hit the pillow. I didn't even have to read her a story."

"I think all the excitement and the football game wiped her out."

"Yeah," he agrees. Then, "You should have let me clean up. You did all the cooking."

"It's not a problem," I tell him.

"Have I told you those cupcakes you made were amazing?"

"Only about ten times."

"Clearly not enough then."

His eyes sparkle, and I feel a pang of attraction in my gut.

I look away and start wiping down the sink.

"You sure I can't do anything to help?" His voice

sounds closer now, deeper, lower, reminding me of long drugging kisses and hot nights in his arms.

"No. I'm all done," I say, but I don't turn around. I'm feeling flustered and heated, and I don't want him to see what I know is written on my face right now—desire.

I hate the effect just his voice can have on me.

"Well then, I guess I'll head off."

"I'll see you out." I pick up the hand towel and dry my hands, taking time to cool down. Then, I turn and follow him out to the front door.

He opens it and steps outside into the night before facing me. He holds the frame with his hand, and my eyes are pulled to his forearm and the veins strongly running through them.

I've traced those veins with my tongue. I've tasted every single part of this man. There isn't a part of his body that I haven't seen, or touched. Or he with mine.

I feel an ache between my legs and press my thighs together.

He wets his lips. "Cam . . . I know I've already said it once today, but thank you for having them all here and making them feel so welcome."

I realize that I'm staring at his mouth, so I lift my gaze to his eyes. "They are welcome anytime." And I mean it.

I've missed being a part of the Kincaids. It felt nice to have that chance again today. And it was even better, knowing that Gigi will have that and them for the rest of her life.

"So, I'll see you tomorrow?" he says.

"You're still picking Gigi up from pre-K? I said I'd work overtime tomorrow."

"Yeah, I was planning on taking her to my place. Thought we could go down to the water, feed the birds. Unless you want me to bring her here?"

"No, it's fine. Take her to yours. She'll love feeding the birds. I can come straight from work and pick her up after I'm finished. I get off at six."

"Don't worry. I'll bring her home at about half past six."

"You sure?"

"Mmhmm."

"Perfect. Thanks, Z."

I smile, and his lip lifts at the corner into that sexy smile of his.

"It's been a hella long time since you called me that."

Shit.

I called him Z.

I used to do that only when I wanted him—sexually, I mean.

I never even realized that was the case until he pointed it out one day. He said that was when he knew I wanted him inside me, which was pretty much all the time.

And, now, I've just called him Z and given myself away. Zeus is nothing if not observant.

My cheeks heat, and I lower my eyes. "Yeah. Weird."

He chuckles softly. "Night, Dove." Then, he leans close and presses his lips to my forehead.

The instant his lips touch my skin, the air between us heightens, like a fully charged lightning rod has just been plunged into the ground beneath us.

I know he feels it, too, because his breaths quicken.

My pulse starts to throb in my neck.

His lips linger for long seconds. I'm about to ask what he's doing even though I'm fully aware of what he's doing, but I know I need to put a stop to it before it gets out of control. But he shifts closer, and my breasts brush his chest, sucking the words out of my head and all the air out of my lungs.

His lips trace a path down my temple, stopping to press a soft kiss to my cheekbone and then my jaw. He keeps kissing until he reaches the corner of my mouth.

My eyes are closed. I open them and find myself staring into his. I know that look. I used to love that look.

"Z . . ." I whisper.

And that's all it takes.

His mouth crashes onto mine.

I open up for him without hesitation. His tongue sweeps inside, sliding against mine, and all rational thought abandons me.

His hands drag up the material of my long dress to my thighs. He lifts me like I weigh nothing.

To Zeus, I don't. The guy is about two hundred fifty pounds of pure, solid muscle, and he squats two hundred kilograms for fun.

My long legs wrap around his waist.

I'm vaguely aware of movement.

Then, the front door bangs shut.

A second later, my back hits the hallway wall.

And that's when things get hot and wild.

We start going at it like we've been starved of each other.

We have.

Five years of pent-up emotions are pouring out into this one kiss.

It's desperate and needy.

And I can't get enough . . . be close enough.

I writhe against him. My fingers driving into his hair. I grip the strands, pulling.

He groans into my mouth, making me smile with the power I have over him.

I take his lower lip between my teeth and sink them in.

He hisses a sound I've missed hearing.

I meet his sex-heated eyes as I lick away the sting with my tongue.

His fingers bite into my ass, and he kisses a path down my neck to the swell of my breasts.

We're covered by a thick sexual fog, and I can't see anything outside of it.

All I can see is him.

All I want is him.

His hips press into mine. I can feel him, hot and hard, through the material of my panties, and I moan, loud.

"Shh, Dove. We have to be quiet."

Gigi.

And that's the bump back to earth that I need. Her name is like a bucket of ice water being thrown over me.

I can't do this. I can't risk doing this with him and it ending badly.

I don't want Gigi getting hurt.

Or me.

I can't gamble my heart on Zeus Kincaid again.

"Stop." I push at his chest with my hand.

He pulls back, looking confused. I slide my legs to the floor.

"Dove?"

"I can't do this with you."

His confusion turns to hurt. I see it sear into his eyes.

He steps back. Drives his fingers into his hair, linking his hands over his head.

"Cam—"

"I need you to leave."

He stares at me for a long moment until I can no longer take it. I look away, eyes staring down the hall.

The next thing I hear is the door being yanked open. I feel the cool of the night air hit my skin. The door closes firmly.

I lean back against the wall.

He's gone.

That's what I wanted, right? That's what I told him to do.

Even still, tears fill my eyes.

And, when I hear his car engine come to life, something ignites inside me. I don't want to put a name to the feeling, but I know it well.

Then, I'm moving. I yank open the front door with no clue as to what I'm going to say to him, only knowing I don't want him to leave like this.

But I'm too late.

His car is already gone.

Chapter Twenty

WORKING OVERTIME WHILE FUNCTIONING on a few hours' sleep is not good. I feel like a zombie.

I forgot how hard it was to do a day's work on little sleep. It's been a while since I had to do it because Gigi started sleeping through the night like the awesome kid she is by the time she was one.

Nothing gets in the way of my girl and her sleep.

Unfortunately for me, plenty was getting in the way of my sleep.

Well, just one thing.

Zeus.

Every time I closed my eyes, I could feel the ghost of his lips on mine and the heat of his body pressed up against me . . . and the hurt in his eyes when I rejected him.

I royally screwed up last night.

I should've headed him off at the pass. But I had been weak, and I'd let him kiss me.

Hell, I'd pretty much attacked his mouth the second he kissed me.

I haven't spoken to him since last night. I received a perfunctory text from him earlier, telling me that he'd picked up Gigi from pre-K and they were at his place.

I could feel the chill emanating from my phone.

I felt sick, reading it.

I still feel sick, and awful and sad.

Kissing Zeus last night only served to remind me of how good things used to be between us. How hot we used to be for each other. How amazing he always made me feel. How easy things between us were back when we were younger and in love.

Now, nothing's easy when it comes to Zeus and me.

I know I need to talk to him about last night. Clear the air between us.

But the chickenshit in me just wants to avoid it.

But I can't avoid him.

He'll be dropping Gigi off later.

So, I'm just going to have to put on my big-girl panties, woman up, and talk to him like a grown-up.

I can do it.

I think.

Ugh.

I just need coffee, and the weak stuff in the station's machine just isn't going to cut it.

I push my desk chair out and lock my computer down.

I'll make a quick run to the coffee shop. I'm due for a break anyway.

I grab my purse and head out of the building.

"Cam," a familiar voice calls.

I turn, seeing Rich. He's dressed in jeans and a T-shirt, a sports bag thrown over his shoulder. He must've just finished a shift.

"Hey." I smile, watching as he jogs down the station steps, coming toward me.

"Hey, stranger," he says when he reaches me.

I haven't seen Rich since our failed night out. Not because I've been avoiding him. We just haven't crossed paths at work. We've texted a few times. Well, he's texted me, asking how I'm doing, and I've replied, but nothing beyond that. He's respecting that I have a lot going on in my life right now, and I appreciate that more than he could know.

"You just getting off?" he asks.

"No." I shake my head. "I said I'd work an extra few hours to catch up on the backlog of paperwork we've got, but I needed coffee, and the station's machine sucks."

"You know the captain does that to get confessions quicker, right? Make the coffee taste like shit and give it to the perps. One sip of that, and they're begging to tell us the truth just so we'll make it stop."

He grins, and I chuckle.

"So, that's why we have a high confession rate." I play along, slapping my hand to my forehead.

"But you can't tell anyone." He lowers his voice. "It's our little secret."

"Gotcha." I pretend to lock up my lips, and he laughs.

"Hell, I've missed you, Cam."

"I've missed you, Dove." Zeus's voice echoes in my head.

My heart reacts to the memory of that and not the words Rich just spoke.

"Well, I'm very missable." I shrug, playing it off, desperate to ignore my internal discomfort.

He smiles again and shoves his hand through his hair.

"I should get going." I thumb over my shoulder. "Can't be gone too long."

"I'll come with you. I could do with a coffee after the long shift I just had."

We walk side by side, making small talk, as we head to the coffee shop.

We reach the door, and Rich is pulling it open when I hear, "Mommy!"

My eyes dart up, and I see Gigi and Zeus walking toward us. She's sitting up on his shoulders, sucking on a Popsicle.

My eyes dart to Zeus's, and the look in them makes me want to shrink and disappear.

"Hey, Gigi girl." I smile up at her even though Zeus's eyes are burning into my skin. "Whatcha doing here?"

"I's wanted a *gurger*."

A *gurger* is a burger. Gigi's called them that forever. The first time she said it, it was so adorable that we've just called them gurgers ever since.

"And Daddy didn't have any in his *fwidge*, so he *bwought* me out to get one. Hey, *Wich*." She waves at him before sticking her Popsicle back in her mouth.

I'm feeling so off-balance at the appearance of Zeus, I don't even comment on the fact that she's eating a Popsicle before having a gurger.

"Hey, Gigi," Rich says to her. "How are you doing?"

"I's good. You wan' some of my Popsicle?" She holds it out to him.

"No, I'm good, but thanks. Zeus, good to see you again."

"I thought you were at work." That's Zeus speaking

to me. He doesn't even bother to acknowledge Rich, which is beyond rude.

I pull my narrowed eyes to him and say, "I am. I just popped out for a coffee and bumped into Rich."

"Convenient. Well, enjoy your coffee," he grinds out. "Say bye to your mom, Gigi."

"Bye, Mommy."

"Bye, baby." I wave at her, but Zeus has already taken off and is striding down the street, away from me.

I stare after them.

Convenient. What the hell is that supposed to mean? Convenient that I was here with Rich?

"Cam?" Rich interrupts my thoughts.

"Mmhmm?"

"You still want that coffee?" he asks.

When I look up, he's holding open the door to the coffee shop.

"Sure," I say.

I cast one more glance in Zeus's and Gigi's direction, my heart giving a painful squeeze, before stepping inside the coffee shop.

Chapter Twenty-One

I'M STARING AT MY computer screen, not actually able to take in a word of the document that I'm correcting, sipping on a triple-shot latte, after yet another crappy night's sleep, courtesy of—yep, you guessed it—Zeus Kincaid.

He was a total ass to me last night when he dropped Gigi off after I got home from work.

I know he was pissed about seeing me with Rich. I'm pretty sure he thinks I arranged to meet Rich for coffee. Even if I had, it's none of his damn business. But, even still, I felt shitty about it. I hated that he thought I would arrange to meet Rich after our kiss the night before.

And I still need to talk to him about that, too.

The list of things that Zeus and I need to discuss is just mounting up.

But, when I did the grown-up thing last night and asked him if we could talk, I got . . . well, figuratively knocked out of the ring.

*

"Zeus . . . do you have a minute to talk?" I asked when he arrived to drop Gigi off.

"No," he said without even looking at me. He leaned down and kissed the top of Gigi's head. "I'll see you tomorrow, baby girl. Love you."

"Bye, Daddy. Wuv you, too."

Then, he turned on his heel and walked back down the driveway. He got in his car and drove away without a backward glance.

And I was left standing there, feeling like a complete and utter tool.

"No."

That was it.

Just no.

Not, *I gotta be somewhere right now, but we can talk later.* Or, *I'm not in the mood to talk right now, Cam.* Even, *I'm pissed at you, and I don't want to talk*, would have been better. Well, not better. But a hell of an improvement on, "No."

Not going to lie; it stung like a bitch when he said that. And, afterward, the more I thought about it, I started to feel a little annoyed. Okay, a lot annoyed.

I drain off my coffee and toss the paper cup in the trash.

Still feeling like death on legs, I grab some change from my purse and make my way to the vending machine to grab some chocolate in the hopes that the sugar might perk me up.

I'm walking down the hall toward the machine when I see Rich coming toward me. If I didn't know better, I'd say, from the expression on his face, I'm the last person on earth he wants to see today.

But I'm not paranoid, so I won't think that at all.

Okay, maybe I'll think it a little.

"Hey, twice in two days. People will start to talk," I gibe. Then, I realize what an awful gag that was in the current situation. You know, the guy I used to occasionally have sex with but stopped when the ex-love of my life and father of my child made a reappearance.

Lame, Cam. Real lame.

Rich smiles as he comes to a stop in front of me, but it's a weak smile. Can't say I blame him after that.

"Sorry." I wince. "That was terrible. Scratch it from your memory. My brain's not functioning properly today. I didn't sleep well last night."

"Why? Have you spoken to Zeus?" he blurts out of nowhere.

That gets my attention straightaway, triggering my internal bat signal to start flashing at a steady pace.

"Not since he dropped Gigi home last night. Why?" I question, my suspicion rising.

"No reason. Just wondered." He tries to give a casual shrug and fails.

"Rich, what's going on?"

He lets out a tired-sounding sigh. "Look, I know you and I aren't"—his eyes convey the word he doesn't want to say out loud in the station hallway where any ears could hear it—"at the moment and that we're currently just friends. But I want to be straight with you. I like you, Cam. And I already wanted more from you . . . before Zeus turned back up in your life. I wanted to be with you. And I won't deny that I was disappointed when you asked for us to slow things down . . . well, to stop doing *that* and just be friends until it calmed down for you with Zeus and Gigi. But I was still hoping that, going forward, we'd come back together and make a go of things. But, now, after thinking things through, I really think it would be best if we just stayed friends."

Hang on. Am I getting dumped by the guy I am no longer sleeping with?

Well, if that's not a knock to the ego, I don't know what is.

"Okay . . ." I say, still feeling a tad confused by his ramblings.

Rich exhales a relieved sound. And my bat signal ramps up to speedy flashes.

"Great. Well, I'm glad we had this little chat. I'll see you around, Cam."

He makes to move past me, and I stop him with my hand on his arm.

"Rich, before you go . . . why did you ask me if I'd spoken to Zeus?"

"Did I?"

"Yes."

He doesn't say anything, but I can see his brain working behind his eyes. He's weighing up the situation, figuring out what to do next, like any good cop would.

But I was raised by a badass cop who never stops digging until she gets the answer she was looking for.

"Rich . . ." I press, using my mom voice, the one I use on Gigi to get her to fess up when I know she's done something wrong.

He lifts a hand to his head and runs his fingers through his hair, scratching at his head. "Look, I wasn't going to say anything because I didn't want to be *that* guy."

"Honestly, I'll settle for you being the guy who tells me what the heck is going on."

He pauses for the longest time, and I'm getting close to tapping my foot with impatience when he says, "I had a visitor last night."

"And?"

"It was Zeus."

Oh.

Fuck.

"What did he say? And how the hell does he know where you live?"

"That was the first question I asked him. Not that I got an answer," he huffs, sounding aggrieved.

Classic Zeus. Doesn't like the question, doesn't give an answer.

"What did he do?"

"Nothing."

My eyes scan his face, looking for any signs of injury. I can't see a mark on him, but that doesn't mean Zeus didn't do anything.

"He didn't hit you, did he?"

"No." Rich laughs loudly, but it sounds too pitchy to be real. "If the guy had hit me, he would've spent the night in a cell here and would've been on his way to a court hearing first thing this morning."

Well, actually, you'd probably still be unconscious right now if he had hit you.

But, of course, I don't say that.

Even still, I am relieved. The last thing I want is Zeus getting arrested for hitting a police officer. And, of course, I don't want Rich getting hit by a guy who could bench-press him using just one arm.

"Did he . . . threaten you?" I ask, half-closing my eyes as I wait for the answer.

"No . . . the guy's not stupid. He's not going to threaten a police officer."

"So, what exactly did he say?"

"Well . . . he said . . ."

Chapter Twenty-Two

"You told Rich that he's standing in the way of my happiness?" I yell the second Zeus opens his front door.

"Hello to you, too, Cam."

"Don't be smart right now. I'm not in the mood."

"Clearly."

"I'm so fucking mad at you."

"I'm getting that." He widens the door, standing aside. "Would you like to come in and be mad at me or stay out there while you yell at me?"

"You're an asshole." I narrow my eyes and stomp past him, stopping just inside.

He closes the door. "Where's Gigi?" he asks.

I give him a less than amused look. "With Aunt Elle. What the hell did you think you were doing, turning up at Rich's house like that?"

"Fighting for my family. Fighting for you."

Well, hell.

"I just didn't expect him to go crying to you."

"He didn't come crying to me. I had to force it out of him."

"You can do better than that guy, Dove. He's got no backbone."

"Better like you, you mean?"

"Well, if you're asking . . ."

"Been there before. Didn't work out so well for me the last time. And, for your information, I'm not even seeing Rich anymore. I haven't been since you came back. He's just a friend."

"Sure he is, Cam. So, you *accidentally* bumped into each other yesterday and decided to go for coffee?"

"Yes! You big jerk! And, if you'd bothered to stay and talk to me last night, then you would have heard me telling you that I'd popped out of work to grab a coffee and bumped into Rich coming out of the station after his shift. We talked briefly. I said I had to go grab my coffee. He said he wanted one—"

"I bet he did."

I glare at him. "He said he wanted coffee, too. So, we walked the few minutes to the coffee shop where I bumped into you and Gigi."

"And that was it?"

"Yes, that was it. We got our coffees. I went back to work, and he went wherever he went—home presumably."

He's staring at me like he's trying to read my thoughts. Then, he sighs and scrubs his hands over his face.

"Just seeing you with him after last night . . . it blind-sided me. It fucking hurt, Dove."

"Zeus . . . last night . . . it was a mistake."

"No, the only mistake I ever made was walking away from you."

"I told you to go."

"I'm not talking about last night."

His eyes bore into mine. His stare is so intense, I can barely handle it.

I look away. "You can't behave like this, Zeus. Going to Rich's, testosterone-filled and pissing on me like you own me."

"You are mine."

Well, if that doesn't just set me off again.

"I'm not yours." I grit my teeth.

"You've been mine since the moment I saw you. That's never going to change."

"God! You're unbelievable." I throw my hands up in the air. "You think the alpha-caveman act is going to work? Well, I'm telling you, it's not!"

"You said you wanted me to fight for you, Cam. Well, this is me fighting in the only way I know how." He spreads his arms out wide.

"Yeah, well, this isn't the way."

"So, tell me what the way is, and I'll do it. I'll do anything to make this work."

"I don't know." I look to the ground. "All I do know is that I don't trust you with my feelings."

"I won't hurt you again," he whispers.

"You once told me that you would never hurt me. So, saying you won't hurt me again carries no weight at all."

"I'm not leaving, Cam."

"You said that before as well. And then I didn't see you for five years."

He drags his hand over his hair, letting out a sound of

frustration. "I explained that. I told you that I was trying to do what I thought was the right thing at the time. But I got it wrong, and it cost me you and four years of my daughter's life. I've paid the price, Cam. But I'm here now. I want to be with you. I want us to be a family."

"You want me because of Gigi."

"Is that really what you think?"

I hold his stare. "I think you love our daughter and that you're telling yourself that you still love me because you so desperately want to get back the time you lost with her."

"I don't have to be with you to spend time with my daughter. I think I've proven that over this past month. And I think you're forgetting that I came back here for you before I even knew about Gigi. I came that morning for you. And, even if there was no Gigi, I would still be here, fighting for you."

"Until you're not."

"I'm not going anywhere! How many times do I have to say this until it sinks in with you? I'm doing everything I can to prove it. I've postponed my fight. I'm renting this place. I'm with you and Gigi every day. I don't know what the hell else I can do to show you that I'm sorry. That I love you."

He's breathing heavily, his eyes frustrated and desperate.

I stare at him, feeling everything and knowing nothing. "I don't know," I whisper, my eyes starting to water under the pressure of my own warring emotions. "I don't know what will fix it." I sigh, my eyes going to the door. "I should go."

"No." He catches my chin in his hand, turning my

eyes to his. "You're gonna stay here, and we're going to figure this out together because I want you, Dove. And I will do anything to make that happen. There's no room for error when it comes to you. I have to get this right with you because I don't want to raise my daughter alongside you while watching another man take you to his bed."

"Zeus . . ."

"You're mine, Dove. You always have been. You always will be."

"But that's just it. I'm not yours! You saw to that when you left me!"

"Cam . . . you have to start forgiving me, or this will never work."

"Maybe I don't want it to work between us. You ever think of that?" I fold my arms over my chest.

"Stop lying to yourself, Cam. The sooner you admit that you still love me, the sooner we can stop messing around and be together."

"Fuck you!" I toss the words at him and make a grab for the door handle.

But he's quicker.

The next thing I know, my back is against the door, my arms pinned over my head.

"Oh no, you don't. You're not walking away from this, Cam. I told you before. We need to work this out once and for all. I've pussyfooted around you for long enough. Now, we work it out. What will it take for you to trust me again?"

"I'll never trust you again. Now, let me go," I grit out.

"You can. And you will. Because you still love me."

I let out a bitter laugh. "So sure of yourself."

"No, Dove. I'm sure of you. I know you better than you know yourself."

"Go to hell."

"Already been there for the last five years. Not looking to go back. Now, tell me you love me, Dove."

"I hate you," I seethe. Hate him and me and everything *us* in this moment.

"Now, we're getting somewhere."

"Are you insane? I just told you I hate you, and you think that's us getting somewhere?"

"Hate is the closest emotion to love. There's a fine line between the two. So, the fact that you say you hate me tells me that your feelings for me are still in there."

"You're wrong."

He's right.

"So, tell me that you don't love me anymore and mean it, Dove. You do that, and I'll never bother you again. I'll be there for Gigi. But I'll leave you alone, so you can get on with your life."

I part my lips to speak.

Say it, Cam. Just say the words, and he'll leave you alone.

"I . . ."

Why can't I say it?

Because you still love him, you idiot. You've always loved him.

I squeeze my eyes shut. Frustration pricking at them.

"I . . . can't," I whisper, defeated.

"That's what I thought," he says low.

The next thing I know, his mouth is covering mine, and for the second time in two days, Zeus is kissing me.

Chapter Twenty-Three

We're hands and lips, tongues and teeth. Heated, crazy, out-of-control lust.

And zero common sense.

Well, me at least.

A voice in the back of my head is yelling that this is a bad idea.

I hit the mute button on that and just focus on touch and taste and need.

Zeus's touch.

His taste.

And my need for him.

It's raging. Wild. Burning like an inferno.

We crash into the wall.

He pushes my skirt up around my hips.

I wrap my leg around his, pressing myself against him, needing to be touching every single part of him.

Just . . . needing him. Right. Fucking. Now.

He growls and grabs hold of my ass, lifting me.

I wrap my legs around his waist.

His tongue plunders my mouth. I match him stroke for stroke.

My fingers wind in his hair and yank.

He chuckles a dark sound against my lips. It's so familiar to me, I could weep.

"You want me to fuck you, Dove?"

I stare at him through heavily lidded eyes. "What do you think?"

He puts his mouth to my ear. Lips grazing my skin. "I think you want me to fuck you against this wall. Hard and deep."

Jesus Christ.

Always so good at the dirty talk.

"Say it. Tell me you want me to fuck you. Tell me how much you want my cock inside you." His hands tighten on me. Fingers biting into my ass.

His eyes come back to mine, and I stare into them. Eyes that are cloudy with lust. For me. Seeing Zeus like this always gave me such a high. Knowing the sexual power I had over him was thrilling.

It still is.

I lean forward and touch my nose to his. My stare on him never wavering. "Stop talking. And just fuck me."

His eyes flash a seductive promise.

I feel his fingers curl into the waistband of my panties. Then, I hear the telltale snap of elastic and feel the thrill-inducing cool air hitting my heated parts.

I don't let him know I like it though. I might want him. But I'm not going easy on him. No way.

"They were my favorite." I scowl at him.

"I'll buy you some new ones."

"Break something. Fix it with money. That how you do things nowadays, Z?"

I know I've hit a nerve from the flare of anger in his eyes. And that excites the hell out of me.

"Tell me you love me," he says through a clenched jaw.

"Fuck you," I bite.

"I will when you say it, Dove." He gently brushes his lips over mine. "Tell me you love me, and I'll give you what you want. My cock deep inside you."

He thrusts up, pressing against my pussy, and I know I've soaked through the material of his shorts.

He chuckles a knowing sound, and it sends fury hurtling through me.

So, I sink my teeth into his bottom lip and bite down hard.

He hisses and pulls back, tongue licking at the wound.

And I get off on the taste of his pain on my tongue.

"You wanna hurt me, Dove?"

Yes. I want to hurt you. And fuck you. And love you . . . and Jesus fucking Christ! I feel like I'm going to explode with all the feelings burning up inside me.

"So, hurt me. Do what you have to. Take what you need."

So, I do.

I curl my hands around the back of his head and yank him back to me.

I kiss him fiercely.

It's rage, and want, and pure unadulterated need.

Teeth clashing. Raw, painful, impassioned kissing.

And he gives it right back to me.

I shove my hands up inside his sweatshirt and rake my nails down his chest.

He pushes up my sweater and yanks down the cup of my bra. Bending his head down, he takes my breast in his mouth.

Teeth dragging over the delicate skin, he bites my nipple at the exact same time that he shoves a thick finger deep inside me from behind.

"Ahh," I moan.

And then another finger before he starts to fuck me with them.

"Always so fucking tight," he groans.

I drag his mouth back up to mine, needing to kiss him more than I need air.

He's fucking me with his hand, his palm slapping against my ass with each penetration of his fingers.

And all I want—*need* to do is come.

I grind my clit against his cock. The friction bringing stars to my eyes.

I hear a sound of pure need and realize it came from me.

Then, I hear an animalistic growl and know that came from Zeus.

His fingers pull out of me.

I whimper at the loss.

He shoves his shorts down his hips.

His cock, erect, long, and incredibly thick, presses against my thigh.

I can feel his pre-cum wet against my skin.

"Say it, Dove. Tell me you love me."

Intense eyes on mine are holding me prisoner.

Biting my lip, I shake my head.

He stares at me so intensely and for so long, an ache pierces my heart, spreading out across my chest.

"Zeus . . ."

In one practiced move, he thrusts up and inside me.

"Fuck," he grits out.

My head thuds back against the wall on a strangled cry, eyes shutting against the wave of emotion at having him inside me again.

It's everything. And nothing I should want.

"Look at me."

I can't.

I shake my head.

His hand grabs my chin, forcing my face to his.

I open my eyes to his brilliant blue eyes watching me intently. His cock is buried deep inside me. His body all around me.

It's too much. And not enough.

"Say it."

I clench my jaw. "I can't." My voice wavers on the words.

His expression shifts into something fiery. "Then, I'll just fuck you until you can."

He pulls out to the tip and then slams back inside me.

Needy lips find mine, passionately kissing me. Desperate hands grip my hips, fingers biting into my skin, as he screws me against the wall.

Long, deep thrusts over and over, his body knowing how to bring mine to the brink. Working me up to the point of mindless desperation. But not giving me what I want. What I need.

"Please, Z . . ." I whimper.

"You want to come?"

"Yes," I breathe.

In and out. Fucking me relentlessly. He tilts his hips a fraction, and—*oh my God* . . .

"That's it," I moan. "Please, don't stop."

His teeth sink into my neck. "Never."

His mouth comes back to mine, and I kiss him desperately sucking on his tongue. His thrusts come quicker, and I know he's as close as I am.

"Tell me you're mine," he growls against my lips.

The urgency in his voice loosens mine. "I'm yours."

He groans a sound of sweet relief. I feel it in every orifice of my body.

"I love you," he says between kisses. "So fucking much. I missed you so much."

And that's what tips me over the edge. Muscles tightening, body spasming, mind numbing, I come around Zeus's cock, triggering his orgasm.

Hips jerking against mine, muffled curses moaned against my mouth. He comes long and hard inside me.

Then, we're just chasing breaths, slowly making our return to reality.

The reality where we're just two people who used to be together.

And who just had sex against his hallway wall.

Christ.

We had sex.

And it was amazing, and I enjoyed it. More than enjoyed it. I loved it.

And . . . I want to do it again.

Nope. No way, Cam. This guy hurt you like no one ever has before.

And Gigi—you have to think of her.

The mere thought of her name brings every reason I had not to do this with him, all of which I chose to ignore, screaming back at me. And finally slapping the sense into me that I so needed ten minutes ago.

"Shit," I whisper.

He must hear it in the tone of my voice because worried blue eyes lift to mine. "Cam?"

"This was a mistake." I drop my legs from around him and shove at him to let me go.

He slips out of me. And I hate the emptiness he leaves behind.

Tears start to burn my eyes from out of nowhere. Not wanting him to see, I quickly sidestep him and start righting my clothes. Covering my breasts up and yanking my skirt back down into place.

I hear the rustle of his clothes as he covers himself behind me.

I catch sight of my torn panties on the floor.

Seeing them there, discarded and used, reminds me of how Zeus once made me feel like that.

And that makes me feel weak and incredibly angry with myself. And him.

I feel a warm trickle on my inner thigh.

It takes my underused brain a good few seconds to register what it is.

Then . . .

Fuck.

"We didn't use a condom," I fire out, whirling around on him.

Surprise flickers in his eyes. Either he didn't realize it either or he wasn't expecting me to say that.

"If you're worried about getting pregnant—"

"I'm not," I snap. "I'm on the pill. Actually, I was on the pill the last time I got pregnant with you, and we weren't using condoms then either, so maybe I should be worried."

Fuck. Fuck. Fuck!

"I'm not worried."

That makes me pause.

He steps forward, closer to me. His expression softening. Eyes warm on me. But all I feel is a chill.

"I can't think of anything I'd want more than to have another kid with you. Except for maybe you and Gigi to come live with me, so we can finally be a family."

"Nope." I step back, bumping into the wall. "No fucking way, Zeus." I'm shaking my head as my back slides along the wall, one hand creeping toward the door. "Don't you dare do this."

"What?" He's following me with his eyes and body. "Tell you that I love you? That I want my girls living with me? That I want my family? Is that so fucking bad, Dove?"

"It's not happening." I curl my fingers around the door handle, gripping it. "This was a mistake. It shouldn't have happened. It won't happen again."

I'm trembling inside. Weak and running scared, and he knows it.

If there's one thing Zeus is good at, it's sniffing out weakness in his opponent.

And I stink of it.

He takes a step closer. "I want you in my bed every night, Dove. My cock buried deep inside you, making love to you." Another step. And another until he's up close against me. "I want more kids with you. I want to see you carrying my baby inside of you. I want my ring on your finger."

I squeeze my eyes shut against all the words he's saying. The words I wanted to hear from him five years ago.

But it's too late now. Too much has happened. I'm not that girl anymore. And I have Gigi to think about.

If Zeus and I got back together and it didn't work out, it wouldn't only hurt me. It'd hurt Gigi.

And if he disappeared on me again, like last time . . .

I can't do that to her. I can't risk it.

I might still love him. I clearly still want him.

But, I don't trust him.

And, without that, we have nothing.

I open my eyes and glare up at him. "No."

"No?" he echoes.

"We're not getting back together. Yes, we had sex. But, that was because we had unfinished business. We never theoretically got to say good-bye, and now, we've done that. So . . . our business is concluded."

His expression is incredulous. "Do you hear yourself right now?"

"Loud and clear." I frown.

"Then, you know that you're talking complete horseshit."

"Fuck you!" I bite.

"Already have, and I intend on doing it again and again and again—"

"God!" I yell. "I hate you so much!"

"We've already established that as well. Right before you told me to put my cock inside you. See where I'm going with this, Dove?"

"Argh!" I scream.

Years and years' worth of pent-up rage floods my veins, making me see red. I shove both my hands hard against his chest, but the bastard doesn't move an inch.

"I don't want you!"

"Stop lying," he fires back.

"Stop telling me what I think and feel!" I scream at him.

"I'll stop when you stop fucking lying to yourself!" he roars.

Then, it's silent. Only the fading sounds of our fury-filled words are left.

Both of our chests are heaving from the physical and emotional exertion of the ire we feel toward each other.

Then, he whispers my name, and it awakens me to the gravity of our situation.

"I have to go." I turn away from him and press down on the handle.

He stops me with his hand on the door. "Don't go." His voice is soft, filled with the sweetest agony.

I feel his firm chest pressing gently against my back. His racing heart is pounding through his chest, trying to reach me. His warm breath is blowing through my hair.

"Stay. *Please*," he whispers.

I want to.

It would be so easy to fall into him again.

But I can't.

So, I close my eyes and let myself feel the pain I endured when he left me. How broken I was. How *he* broke me.

And then I think about how much I love my daughter.

And that's enough to help me steel myself against him.

I seal my heart off, open my eyes, and look back to him. "I have to go. Gigi is waiting for me."

His throat moves on a swallow. Indecision fills his eyes.

Then, he moves his hand away from the door and steps back, giving me the space to leave.

I exhale, pull open the door, and step outside.

The freshness of the air hitting my face does nothing to clear my head.

"Cam . . ."

I stop, but I don't turn around. If I do, I'll crumble.

I hear him move closer.

Feel the warmth of him when he's near.

My heart starts to feel . . . to ache.

I shut my eyes again, desperately fighting against my feelings.

"Cam . . ." he says again, his voice deep and thick with emotion. "Just because I'm letting you go . . . doesn't mean I'm letting *you* go."

The understanding of his words whispers through me, heading straight for my weakening heart, repairing and breaking it, all at the same time.

"I fucking love you. I've loved you since I was seventeen years old and saw you standing at the fair, looking like the answer to a question I didn't know I'd asked. I knew it then, and I still know it now. There is no one else for me. I'm yours. And you sure as hell are mine. We're meant to be together. And the more you fight me on this, the more I'll fight back, and twice as hard. And I'll fight dirty if I have to. For as long as necessary. I'm here and ready to do this to get you back with me, where you belong. I've never lost a fight, Dove. And

I don't intend on losing this one. You're far too fucking important to me for that to happen."

I pull in a shuddering breath. My heart hammering in my chest. Thoughts and feelings pulling me in two very different directions.

I don't say anything. I *can't* say anything.

I mean, what can I say to that?

So, I do the only thing I can right now. I take a step forward, away from him, and then another and another. And I keep moving until I'm inside my car and driving away from him.

But, deep down, I know it doesn't matter how much distance I put between myself and Zeus because I've always been weak when it comes to him.

Even now, I can hear his words in my head, smell his scent on my skin . . . feel his body against mine.

And I crave these things. Like an addict.

Maybe I have more of my mother inside me than I realized.

Knowing that and knowing Zeus and how he is when he wants something, it means I'm screwed.

Because me against him . . . it's like a gazelle going up against a lion.

I won't survive.

I know it. And he knows it.

So, there's only one thing I can do.

Avoid him like the plague.

Chapter Twenty-Four

AVOIDING SOMEONE WHEN YOU have a kid together is as difficult as you think it would be.

It's been a week since The Mistake, as I'm referring to it.

Saying I had sex—amazing, soul-searing, body-shivering sex—with Zeus has me saying stupid shit like that and making me want to turn up at his place and do it all over again.

So, yeah, The Mistake, it is.

Dodging Zeus is exhausting.

And I'm ashamed to say that I've used my daughter as an aid for avoidance. I'm a terrible mother. But, whenever Zeus and I have had to be together in the same room because of Gigi, I've made sure to follow my four-year-old daughter around like a shadow at all times.

I'm pathetic and weak.

Aunt Elle has been amazing.

After The Mistake, I drove straight home. Pretended like everything was okay. Then, after putting Gigi to bed, I fell apart. I literally cried on Aunt Elle's shoulder.

She didn't pass judgment. She just listened to me.

Then, she asked me what I wanted. And she said, if that was Zeus, then it was okay. It wasn't something to be ashamed of because we love who we love. Or as it said in Selena Gomez's song, "The Heart Wants What It Wants."

I didn't pretend to Aunt Elle and say I didn't love him still. Because what would be the point? I've loved Zeus since I was fifteen.

Five years of his absence didn't change that. So, at this point, I don't think anything will.

I know I'll always love him.

But trust him?

His word counts for nothing with me. And I don't know if it ever will again.

The only thing I do trust is his love for Gigi. I know he'd never willingly hurt her.

But he doesn't see what I do.

If Zeus and I got back together, Gigi would get attached to us as a family. And, if Zeus and I didn't work out, it would hurt her. I won't do that to her.

I won't do that to myself.

No matter how much I love him.

I told all of this to Aunt Elle.

She told me that she loves me. That she's proud of me. And that she'll support whatever decision I make.

But there's no decision to make.

I've already made it.

Zeus and I are never happening. Despite his claims that we're inevitable, and his promise to fight until he has me back.

All I need is some time. Just enough to strengthen myself against him. A few more weeks, and I'll be fine.

Or that's what I've been telling myself anyway.

I've managed a week already. Okay, it's been hard, and he's tried his best to get me alone, but I've succeeded in not letting it happen once.

He's here every night with Gigi, putting her to bed and reading her a bedtime story. And, when he's done, if Aunt Elle's not here to act as a buffer and it's just me and him, then I'm conveniently in the shower or bath.

So, he leaves.

But then, without fail, about an hour later, he calls my cell.

And, each time, I don't answer.

He leaves a voice message. The same message every time.

"I'm not giving up, Dove. I love you."

Then, I spend the rest of the night pretending like I don't care while intermittently listening to the message—sometimes crying, sometimes drowning my sorrows in a bar of chocolate.

Then, I delete the voicemail. And go to bed.

And the cycle starts all over again the next day.

But I can do this. I will do this.

He will realize I'm not going to break. That The Mistake was just that, and we're never getting back together—cue Taylor Swift's song.

And the cycle will break.

It has to.

Because I won't risk my daughter's happiness for anything.

I'm rushing around, getting Gigi ready for school and myself ready for work.

Zeus offered to come and pick her up to take her to pre-K, but I declined, knowing that Aunt Elle wouldn't be here and Gigi wouldn't be a good buffer. She's a kid monster in the morning, and her sole ambition in life is to glue her eyes to the television and ignore everything I ask her to do.

I'm in the kitchen, making our lunches—peanut butter and jelly sandwiches for us both. I might be twenty-four, but I have the palate of a child—when the doorbell rings.

I pause as an excited chill creeps down my spine.

Excited at the thought that it could be Zeus.

Chilled at the thought that it could be Zeus.

Messed up, thy name is Cameron.

"I gots it!" Gigi yells out, sounding a hell of a lot chipper than I feel.

"No, you's don't!" And I've also been picking up on my daughter's vocab. *Awesome*. "What have I told you about answering the door?" I say sternly as I walk out of the kitchen and into the hall.

Gigi has stopped just short of the door with a guilty look on her face.

"That just 'cause it's our doorbell ringing doesn't means we knows who it is."

"That's right, Gigi girl. So, what do you do when the doorbell rings?"

"I's waits for Mommy or Granny Elle. Or Daddy if he's here."

That last bit stabs into my heart like a shard of glass.

"That's right." I smile at her even though it's the last

thing I feel like doing. "So, now that I'm here with you, you can open the door."

Gigi unlocks the door and pulls it open.

"Daddy!" she screams and jumps at him.

Zeus catches her in his arms and holds her close, hugging her. "Morning, baby girl." He kisses her cheek. His eyes drift to me. "Morning, Cam."

"Hi," I say. "What are you doing here?" I try to say it without sounding too accusatory.

"I wanted to see my girl before school."

Gigi slaps her hands to his cheeks and brings his focus to her. "You means, *giwls*, Daddy. You wants to see Mommy before work, too, right?"

"Right." He smiles at her. Then, his eyes move to mine. "I always want to see your mom." The wanting look in his eyes makes my heart go kaboom.

Welp.

"Also, I got you something," he tells Gigi, moving his stare back to her.

"You dids?" she squeaks.

"A surprise," he whispers.

"I *woves* surprises!" Gigi exclaims. "What is it?"

Zeus looks at me. "Am I okay to come in for a minute?"

I glance at the clock on the wall. "We've got only a few minutes," I tell him.

"That's all I need."

He puts Gigi down and walks into the hall with her glued to his side. I shut the door behind them and lean up against it.

Then, he pulls an envelope out from the pocket of his biker jacket, gets down to his knee, and hands it to Gigi.

"You gots me a *wetter*, Daddy?"

His lips tilt into that devastating smile of his. "Kinda. Open it," he urges.

Intrigued, I step closer.

Gigi rips open the envelope, dropping it to the floor. There's a folded piece of paper inside.

Gigi opens the paper, and something that looks like tickets flutter to the floor.

Zeus quickly picks them up.

"What's it say, Gigi girl?" I ask her.

"It's a picture of *Sweeping Bweauty's* castle, Mommy." She turns the picture to me.

Huh?

Zeus hands the tickets to her. "And what are these, Gigi girl?"

She frowns in concentration. "I dunnos, Daddy."

"They're tickets," he says. "And who's that right there?" He points at something on the tickets.

"Mickey Mouse," Gigi answers without hesitation.

"And where would you find Mickey Mouse and Sleeping Beauty's castle?"

"Disney World," I whisper at the same time as Gigi screams, "Disney World!"

"That's right, baby girl." He beams at her. "I got us tickets to go to Disney World this coming weekend."

This weekend?

"You dids?"

"I did."

"You's the best Daddy ever!"

She launches herself at him, and he catches her, chuckling as she wraps her arms around his neck.

And I start to feel sick.

He's taking her to Disney. I've never been able to afford that.

And it's all the way across the country. Meaning he's going to be taking her away from me. I've never spent a night away from Gigi since the moment she was born.

"Mommy! Looks!" She disentangles herself from Zeus and dashes to me. "We's going to Disney! I gonna gets to see Flynn *Wider*! I's can tell him we gets married when I's a big girl. I gonna need my *pwettiest* dress, Mommy! I can't wait to tell Granny Elle!"

She's bouncing off the wall with excitement, and I'm smiling big for her, but inside, I'm sinking.

"That's great news, Gigi girl. I'm super happy for you." I bend down and hug her. "Would you do me a favor? Go grab your reading book from your room for me. We need to take it back to pre-K today."

"Okay, Mommy!" She runs off, up the stairs, singing "When Will My Life Begin" from the *Tangled* movie.

My eyes meet Zeus, who's now standing across from me.

"You should have talked to me first," I say quietly, an edge to my voice. "You can't just go off and book a vacation without consulting me."

"It's just a few days in Disney World. And I would've run it past you, but I haven't been able to get five minutes alone to speak to you."

He's got me there. But still . . .

"Look, I'm not trying to be a bitch or be awkward, Zeus. It's just . . ."

"What?"

"I've never been away from Gigi," I admit. "I haven't

spent a night away from her since the moment she was born."

His expression turns tender. "There are three tickets, Dove."

"What?"

"I booked it for *you*, me, and Gigi to all go together."

"Oh." *Oh*. "Hang on. You've booked this for me, too?"

Well, if that doesn't just annoy the crap out of me.

He nods, eyes carefully watching me.

"And it's for this weekend?"

"Three nights actually. We leave Friday."

"I work Friday." I fold my arms over my chest, feeling somehow wronged that he just went off and did this.

"Not this Friday, you're not."

"Says who?"

"Your boss. I had Elle ask on your behalf for the time off. It's all been arranged."

"Aunt Elle?" I blurt out.

"Yeah. I told her that I wanted to surprise you and Gigi. She was more than happy to help me out, getting you the time off work."

And, apparently, Aunt Elle is now a traitor.

"Gigi has pre-K," I counter.

"It's a few days, Cam." He sighs, clearly frustrated by my reluctance.

My eyes go to the ceiling. Gigi has to go to Disney; otherwise, she'll be devastated if she doesn't. And I don't relish the thought of being away from her for four days and three nights. So, it looks like I'm going to Disney World with them.

"I didn't do this to piss you off," he says gently.

"I just wanted to do something nice for Gigi. I want to spend time with her . . . and you."

"Don't . . ." I warn him, bringing my eyes back to him. "You want me to come with you, then I'll do it on one condition."

"Name it."

"You have to promise to lay off me. No talk about us getting back together while we're at Disney. This vacation is about Gigi. Not you and me."

"Okay," he says. "I won't mention a single thing about you and me the whole time we're there. Scout's honor."

I bark out a laugh. "You, a Boy Scout? Hardly."

He grins. "I'm an honorary member nowadays."

"Sure you are, Zeus."

I laugh again. So does he.

His twinkling eyes catch mine. The moment they lock with mine, they turn serious. My breath halts.

"I miss you," he says in a low voice, moving closer.

My body instantly reacts to him. My nipples harden. His eyes lower to my chest, like he can see them through my bra and shirt.

His eyes come back to mine before roaming down to my mouth. "I can still taste you." His voice is a low growl.

And I lick my lips without conscious thought.

"I can still feel you around my cock, Dove. I can't stop thinking about it . . . me inside you. I've been hard for a week, baby. A whole fucking week."

"Y-you just promised," I stutter, my body trembling with need for him. "You said you'd stop with this."

He leans in and whispers in my ear, "I said I'd stop while we were in Disney World. We're not there yet."

The sound of Gigi bounding down the stairs is a goddamn relief because having him this near had me close to just grabbing him and kissing the hell out of him.

Zeus seamlessly steps back from me. He's instantly calm and collected.

Me . . . well, I'm a jittering jumble of a mess, desperately trying to pull myself back together after he just reduced me to a quivering idiot in a matter of seconds.

Zeus—1.

Cam—0.

"I gots the book, Mommy." She thrusts it at me, and my trembling hand takes it. "Daddy, are we staying in a hotel? Does it have a pool?" she fires up at him.

He picks her up and looks into her face as he talks to her, "We are, baby girl, and yep, it has a pool and a view of the Magic Kingdom." His eyes come to mine. "I got us a suite to stay in. Two bedrooms."

His stare smokes through me, and my insides shake hard. Setting off an incessant throbbing between my legs.

I'm so screwed.

He's got me backed into a corner. The oddest of corners, because, now, I'm wanting the Disney trip to quickly roll around, so I can have a break from Zeus trying to win me back, by being tricked into spending time with him, while sleeping in the same two-bedroom suite as him.

Confused? Yep, me too.

Remember what I said before about me being a gazelle and him a lion?

Yep, well, the lion has just chased me into a dead end, and I didn't even see it coming.

The only saving grace I have is that he's promised

not to talk about us while we're there. And, if he's not talking about us or using his sexiness as a weapon against me, then I'll be fine.

Totally fine.

And, also, Gigi will be with us, and nothing can happen when you've got your four-year-old kid, who's all hopped up on Disney, right?

Chapter Twenty-Five

WRONG.

Zeus might not be saying anything, but the looks he keeps giving me . . . God, the looks alone are enough to do me in.

And I don't know if he's sprayed himself with sex pheromones or if it's just seeing him here with Gigi, doting on her and just being an amazing father, or if it's feeling like we're actually a family unit, but it's setting off explosions in my ovaries and making me horny.

Only I could get turned on while at Disney World.

I'm going straight to hell.

The suite we're staying in is in the Bay Lake Tower hotel, which is right by the Magic Kingdom and overlooks the park. It's beautiful.

And it has two bedrooms.

One for me and Gigi to stay in. The other for Zeus.

He said he tried to get a three-bedroom suite, but there was none available.

But I don't care. Bunking in with my beauty is no problem at all.

It's the beast I have to be careful not to get into bed with.

The other thing we have while we're here is security.

I sometimes forget how famous Zeus is.

It's easy to forget when we're in Port Washington, and it's just us. But, when you come out into the big wide world, especially in a place like Disney, there are always going to be people who recognize him.

Zeus didn't want the security. He said it would only bring attention to him. But Disney insisted on supplying it when they knew who they had staying with them because a famous person in Disney could become a security risk. And, because we would have Gigi with us, Zeus relented immediately.

Her safety is nonnegotiable

And it's not too bad, having security. The two guys assigned to us are Steve and Donovan—who, don't get me wrong, are big guys but nothing like Zeus. He towers over the both of them. But they seem like good guys, and it's nice to have that little extra safety even though I know Zeus wouldn't let anything happen to Gigi or me.

Steve and Donovan stay a close distance behind us, so it's not like they're even really there with us half the time, so we're still getting time together, behaving like every other family here.

Except we're not a family. Not in the real sense.

Your choice, Cam, remember?

Sigh.

The only time Steve and Donovan make their presence known is when people start to approach Zeus, asking for photos and autographs, and then they intervene.

I know people approaching Zeus bothers Gigi. She

doesn't say it, but I can tell. She understandably wants his full attention, and it's frustrating for her when someone tries to take her daddy's focus away from her.

But Zeus isn't letting it happen. He's here for Gigi and no one else.

He hasn't been signing autographs or taking photos with anyone. That's not him being an ass. That's him wanting to have some quality time while on vacation with his daughter, and I admire him for that.

I also admire his ass in the jeans he's wearing today, but that's another story.

The good thing is that Zeus doesn't even have to tell people that he's not willing to take a picture with them. Steve and Donovan do it for him in a polite way, telling them he's on vacation with his family.

That is obviously piquing interest because, as far as the world knows, Zeus is a single man with no family, except for his siblings.

Well, he is a single man.

But whatever.

And he might not be posing for pictures, but people are still taking them.

As I've recently discovered there's an Instagram page called DILFs of Disney. And, of course, Zeus appeared on it the first day we were here. A picture of him with Gigi in his arms. She was dressed in her new Rapunzel outfit that Zeus had bought her, and she was feeling tired, so he picked her up to carry her. He looks seriously hot in the picture. He's only wearing black jeans, sneakers, and a white V-neck T-shirt, but hell fire, he's devastatingly handsome.

There are a lot of comments on the picture. Mostly, people are commenting that they didn't know he had a daughter. *Neither did he until a few months ago.* And maybe it's not his daughter. Maybe it's a friend's child. Then, people are saying they heard he's on vacation with his family.

Maybe we should've thought about what we had Steve and Donovan tell people, but I guess it's too late now.

But I can see the speculation building, and it's honestly making me feel uneasy. Something in my gut doesn't feel right about it. But I'm not going to let it ruin our vacation, so right now, I'm choosing to ignore it and enjoy my time here.

We're currently on Main Street, waiting for the fireworks to start. We didn't go to the fireworks last night, as Gigi was tired from the flight and her first day in Disney, which had consisted of going into every shop and riding every ride possible. She crashed as soon as we got to our room, and so did I. I lay down on the bed with her, and when I opened my eyes again, it was morning.

But we're here to watch them now. It's eleven p.m., and Gigi has never stayed up this late before. She's flagging a little, but she's desperate to see them. And, honestly, I really want to see them, too. So, Zeus has her up on his shoulders, carrying her, and we're standing in the street, waiting for it to start, Steve and Donovan close by.

"Mommy! Daddy! *Wook*!" Gigi points at the light show happening in the sky. "So *pwetty*!" she says.

I smile up at her. "Not as pretty as you," I tell her.

She grins at me before her eyes go back to the sky.

We watch the show, oohing and aahing at the fireworks and music and light show. It's absolutely stunning. And heart-warming.

And it's making me feel all fuzzy inside.

I guess it's the Disney effect.

Gigi is clapping her hands with excitement. When we're halfway through the show, the *Tangled* part comes on. Chinese lantern effects are floating up Sleeping Beauty's castle, and "I See the Light" starts to play. Gigi is practically bouncing on Zeus's shoulders. He has to steady her with one arm banded over his chest, holding her legs there.

"*Tangled*! *Wook*, Mommy! Daddy! It's *Tangled*! 'Punzel and Flynn! I loves Flynn!" She starts to loudly sing along to the song.

I'm smiling up at her when I see Zeus's lips moving along to the song with her.

I grin at him. Big, tough Zeus Kincaid is singing a Disney song. And, inside, I'm melting.

And tired of fighting that I want him.

Zeus catches me watching him. He smiles that beautiful smile of his, and my stomach flips.

My hand moves, unbidden, seeking his.

I find it, warm and strong. I slide my palm against his.

His eyes flicker with surprise.

I keep my eyes on him. Bottom lip caught between my teeth, I push my fingers between his, giving him no doubt of what's on my mind.

His expression changes, becoming dark and serious and wanting.

I'm playing a dangerous game. I know that.

But I want him.
I'm not fighting it anymore tonight.
Tomorrow, I'll go back to fighting.
But, tonight, I'm putting down my gloves.

Chapter Twenty-Six

GIGI IS ASLEEP ON Zeus's shoulders before we even leave Main Street. Steve and Donovan accompany us back to the hotel, seeing us to our suite.

While Zeus carries Gigi to bed, I lock up. I take the bag with Gigi's evening purchases into the living room. That girl is getting spoiled rotten here, but then, if you can't spoil your kid in Disney, where can you spoil them?

Then, I go into the little kitchen area and grab two bottles of beer out of the mini fridge. I pop the caps off them both.

I take a much-needed swig from my bottle before carrying them out into the living room.

I'm not a big drinker, and Zeus rarely drinks due to his training, but I figure we deserve one after a long day of fun.

And I'm not in any way trying to get him drunk, so I can have my wicked way with him. I know I don't need that to get Zeus.

He's made it more than plainly clear that he wants me.

No, this is Dutch courage for me. And I don't want to drink alone.

I put my bottle down next to Zeus's and stand at the window, looking out over the park.

I hear the click of Gigi's bedroom door shutting.

I turn to see him coming into the living room.

"She okay?"

"Out for the count," he says, walking toward me.

"I got you a beer." I indicate to his bottle on the coffee table.

He doesn't acknowledge what I just said. He walks straight past the beer and toward me.

That's when I recognize the look in his eyes. I saw it plenty of times over the years we were together. His hunting look.

My legs start to tremble. My stomach somersaulting.

And, even though I want this . . . him . . . I find myself backing up, pancaking myself to the window.

He reaches me, chest flush against mine. His big hands slide down my thighs, curling around the backs of them, and he lifts me off the floor, forcing me to wrap my legs around his waist and my arms around his neck.

"What are you doing?" I whisper, my voice quietly shaking.

Stupid question. Because I know exactly what he's doing. What I've wanted him to do since we arrived here. What I told him with my actions earlier.

He brings his face closer to mine. "You know exactly what I'm doing. Giving you what we both want." Then, he covers my mouth with his and kisses me.

I immediately open up for him. His mouth is hot

against mine. His tongue slides into my mouth, making me moan.

I press myself closer to him.

He deepens the kiss. A day's worth of stubble is scratching against my skin, turning me on further, reminding me of how it used to feel against the tender skin of my inner thighs.

The thought makes me clench my thighs tighter around him.

I'm needy and wanting him badly.

"Bedroom," I say against his lips. It's all I can manage to say.

Zeus moves us through the space, heading for the room he's been sleeping in, while I devour every inch of skin on his neck.

He carries me into the room and closes the door behind him.

"Does it have a lock?" I ask him.

"No."

"Gigi might wake up and come in."

"Babe, she's not waking up for anything or anybody."

True. When my girl's out, she's out.

"Okay," I breathe. Then, I kiss him again.

He carries me over to the bed, putting me down on the edge of it.

He takes a step back. His eyes roam over me, making me shiver.

"Strip," he says, his voice like gravel.

On command, I reach for the hem of my top and pull it over my head before sense climbs into my brain.

I toss my top to the floor and then say, "Just because

we're doing this, it doesn't mean we're getting back together."

"Mmhmm," is his response.

"Zeus." I frown.

"Dove."

"Say it."

His brows pull together. "It doesn't mean we're getting back together. Satisfied?"

No.

"Yes."

"Good. Now, lift your skirt up and show me that gorgeous pussy of yours."

God, I love it when he talks to me like this. All dirty and domineering.

And, now that we've got the preliminaries out of the way, I'll do whatever he asks me to do.

I part my legs and pull my skirt up.

His eyes darken. "Your panties are blocking my view."

Smiling salaciously, I lift my ass and slip my panties down my legs. I kick them aside.

Fingers on my thighs, I tease my skirt back up, over my hips, and open my legs again, giving him the view he wants. "Satisfied?" I throw his earlier comment back at him.

"Almost . . ." He presses his index finger to his lips. "Spread those legs wider, ballerina." He indicates, using the same finger.

Annoyance rises in my throat. "I'm not a ballerina anymore, remember?"

His jaw tightens. "I remember. Now, spread your legs."

Defiance pokes at me. I open my legs a fraction wider.

Irritation flashes in his eyes.

He walks forward, standing between my legs, and drops down to his knees, so we're at eye-level.

He leans in and puts his mouth against my ear. My breath stutters.

"You can do better than that. Don't forget, I know exactly how flexible you are."

I don't get a chance to tell him that I'm also five years older and that I have had a baby since then. Because, the next thing I know, I'm flat on my back, my legs are spread akimbo, and Zeus's mouth is on my pussy.

And, apparently, I am still *that* flexible.

"God," I breathe.

His eyes lift to mine, his mouth glistening with me. "That's what they say, baby."

"Cocky bastard," I mutter.

"And you know that I definitely have the goods to back that fact up."

I smile despite myself.

But the smile is wiped off a second later, replaced with a muffled cry of pleasure, when he puts his mouth back on me, sucking my clit.

His finger pushes inside me a second later, quickly followed by another, and then he fucks me with them.

I'm writhing with need, needing more . . . needing all of him.

His free hand clamps down over my stomach, holding me in place.

"Play with your tits," he roughly orders me.

He always did like to see me touching myself. Well, when he could get involved, too.

God, I remember the times I would tease him, touching

myself, turning him on to the point of madness, when he couldn't have sex with me because he had a fight the next day and was in abstinence.

After his fight was done though, I would get the hell fucked out of me. Just the way I liked it.

I unclip my bra. Thank God for front fastening.

My hands go to my breasts. Cupping one in each hand, I roll my nipples between my fingers while he mercilessly licks, sucks, and bites my clit.

"Z . . . I'm close . . ." I groan. And boy am I ever.

Zeus is the only one who's ever been able to get me off this quickly. With other men, it's always taken longer.

Maybe it's because he's the one who taught me about my body . . . taught me about sex. He was the first guy I slept with.

I, once upon a long time ago, thought he would be the only guy I'd have sex with.

Turned out, I was wrong. But I won't go down that road of bitterness right now.

Not while he's giving me the incredible pleasure that he is at this moment in time.

His fingers slip out of me, replaced by his tongue. It plunges in me as he fucks me with it.

His thumb presses down on my clit, and like a hot button, I come apart. Every muscle in my body contracting, my clit pulsing, I ride the waves of my orgasm with quiet, muffled curses before I sag, boneless, into the bed.

I feel Zeus move.

I lift my head.

He's standing at the foot of the bed. His erection is straining through his jeans.

The sight of it makes my mouth water.

I sit up on the bed. I slip my bra off my arms and throw it to the floor.

I still have my skirt on. So, I stand up on the bed and shimmy it down my hips. Unzip it and then push it down my legs, ridding myself of my last item of clothing.

Zeus's eyes watch me the whole time.

In all my confidence in the knowledge of how much he wants me, I forgot that this is the first time that Zeus has seen me naked since I had Gigi. We didn't exactly get to the naked part the last time we had sex. We were in too much of a rush to undress.

Not this time though.

And don't get me wrong; I am in good shape, thanks to the dancing. But my stomach is a bit more rounded than it used to be. No six-pack for this mama. And I have some stretch marks. Cellulite on my ass and thighs. And my boobs aren't as perky as they used to be pre-breastfeeding.

"God, Cam," he says roughly. "I didn't think it was possible, but you're even more beautiful now than before. You're impossibly beautiful. I don't deserve you. I never did. But fuck if I don't want you. I'm selfish enough to take whatever you'll give me."

And my momentary lack of confidence is erased by his words and the way he's looking at me.

Like I'm everything.

It thrills and terrifies me.

And that's the problem with us.

I love him. But he hurt me badly. I am terrified to let go in case he does it again.

I speak past the emotion clogging my throat, "This . . . me. Right now . . ." I whisper, "This is what I can give you."

His eyes hold mine, not a flicker of feeling, or response in them.

A beat later, he reaches back and pulls his T-shirt off over his head, dropping it to the floor.

I immediately see it. "You got another tattoo?" I step off the bed, moving closer.

Zeus had one tattoo that I knew of. He's had it for as long as I've known him. It's on his back, covering a large portion of it. It's for his mom. Some of the lyrics from "Amazing Grace," interwoven around each other with angel wings at either side. It's a gorgeous tattoo.

But this tattoo is new, and it's on his chest. His left pec, to be exact. It's a bird in flight. It's . . .

My heart putters to a stop, my eyes flashing up to his.

"Is that a . . ." I can't bring myself to say it.

"A dove. Yes." His eyes carefully watch me.

A multitude of emotions grips me like a hand around my heart. "When did you get it done?" I suddenly feel like I'm talking through cotton wool.

"After the Hagan fight."

"That was a month after we broke up." Around the same time that I found out I was pregnant with Gigi. "Why?" I question.

He exhales roughly. "Because I needed something, Cam. Some connection to you. I had nothing left but memories. I had to let you go, and . . . you on my skin, it was all I could have. I know that probably doesn't make sense—" He doesn't get to finish because I launch myself at him.

My mouth collides with his, and I kiss him desperately.

He tightly wraps his arms around me.

The kiss is out of control. Like the feelings swirling through my body.

I attack his jeans with my hands, needing to feel all of him against every part of me.

My hands are trembling with emotion and excitement. I manage to get the button and zipper undone.

Zeus takes over, quickly removing his jeans along with his boxer shorts.

Then, he's gloriously naked.

God, I've missed him.

Our lips crash back together. Our mouths fusing like we've never kissed before.

We stumble back to the bed. Hands and mouths everywhere.

Somehow, I end up on top of Zeus.

I push up to sit on him. He stares up at me, watching me with those stunning eyes of his.

I rise up onto my knees and take his cock in my hand. Curling my fingers around it, I squeeze hard.

A sound of pleasure hisses between his clenched teeth.

And it empowers me to take what I want right now.

Him.

I position his cock at my entrance. Our eyes locked together, I slowly lower myself down onto him. Inch by thick inch until he's fully seated deep inside me.

The look in his eyes is filled with so much intensity that I can barely take it.

So, breaking the connection, I lean forward and kiss him. I start to move up and down. He threads one hand in my hair, the other gripping my hip, guiding my slow strokes.

As the kisses deepen, the tempo of my body speeds up.

The next thing I know, I'm flipped onto my back, and Zeus is taking over.

He sits back on his haunches. The tip of his cock just inside me.

He reaches back and grabs hold of my legs, pushing them forward until my knees are almost pressed to my chest. He holds them there.

Then, he thrusts his cock back in.

"Ahh," I softly cry out in pleasure as he hits that spot deep within me.

His hands leave my legs and drop to the mattress on either side of my head, and then he starts to fuck me.

I hook my knees over his shoulders as he continues to thrust into me, pounding me with his cock.

Turning his head, he starts to kiss my leg, his tongue stroking the skin, teeth biting, and it feels amazing.

But I know Zeus, and I won't stay here for long. When he fucks like this, he likes to fuck in as many ways as possible.

And I'm right.

I'm moving. Turned over onto my stomach. Ass in the air. Legs spread. And he's back inside me.

Hands gripping my ass cheeks, fingers biting into my skin, he thrusts in and out of me. Skin slapping skin in the most delicious way. The sound turning me on even more.

"Fuck," he grits out. "I missed you so fucking much."

I missed you, too.

His arm comes underneath me, and he lifts me up.

Sitting on his haunches, cock still inside me, he puts me in his lap. My back to his chest.

"Ride me," he whispers roughly into my ear.

So, I do.

With his mouth and tongue on my neck. His hands on my breasts, pinching my nipples. Sweat mists my skin. Slick against his.

One hand leaves my breast and slips between my thighs.

His fingers find my clit, and he starts to tease me to the point of madness.

My legs are shaking. My heart racing.

But I keep fucking him, harder and harder, until I'm coming apart in his arms.

I've barely finished coming when I'm lifted off him, and my back hits the mattress. A second later, Zeus's body hits mine. Another second, and he's back inside me. And, this time, he's not playing.

This is pure, animalistic fucking.

He's gone to the edge, ready to go over. I can see it in his eyes.

He needs this. He needs me.

I hook my legs over his hips, wrapping them around his back. I press my hands to his chest. To his tattoo.

Then, I lean up and place a kiss on it.

He stills.

I lay my head back down. His eyes are on mine, and the look in them makes my heart ache.

He takes my face in his hands and leans down to kiss me.

I wrap my arms around him and kiss him back.

Then, he's moving again.

But, now, it doesn't feel like fucking. It feels an awful lot like making love.

But I can't bring myself to change the point we're at.

I want to be here too much.

I feel my second orgasm start to build quickly.

"You'll come again, Dove." It's not a question. It's a fact.

Zeus knows what he can do to me. Just like I know what I can do to him.

"Yes," I breathe as I score my nails over his shoulders.

He growls and thrusts hard against me, his pelvis hitting me at just the right point.

"Again," I gasp.

And he gives me what I want. And he keeps giving it to me until I'm coming again, and I'm coming hard, squeezing his cock with my inner muscles.

"Fuck . . ." he pants, his head buried in my neck.

A ragged sound escapes him, and I feel him jerk inside me as he starts to come.

We lay here, our uneven breathing the only sound.

Zeus lifts his head from my shoulder. His eyes meeting mine. His stare is smoldering.

He brings his mouth to mine and gently kisses me.

He makes to pull back, but I'm not ready to let him go, so I chase his mouth with mine. Hands sliding up into his hair, I kiss him, telling him with my lips that I don't want to end this moment just yet, and he's more than happy to oblige.

We kiss like teenagers making out for the first time, reminding me of another life.

I allow myself to indulge in it. Until I know it's time to let go.

"I should clean up," I tell him.

He stares down at me for a beat and then says, "Stay there."

When he pulls out of me and goes to the bathroom, it's like the spell is broken. Reality is back with a vengeance. And it's like a cool chill over my skin.

I've just slid my legs over the side of the bed when he appears again in all his naked glory with a cloth in his hand.

He steps up to me and presses it between my legs, cleaning me. Then, he leans down and gives me a soft kiss on the lips.

If he notices that I don't respond to his kiss, he doesn't say anything.

He takes the cloth back to the bathroom. And, this time, when he returns, I'm on my feet, gathering the rest of my clothes from the floor. I've already got my bra and panties back on.

He stops by the bed and stares at me. "Were you even going to say good-bye before you left?" The sarcasm in his voice is evident, and it hits my spine like a hot poker.

"Don't be an ass, Zeus. You knew that us having sex wasn't going to change anything."

"Yeah. But I didn't expect you to fuck and run."

"I'm not fucking and running." I frown. "I'm just going back to my room. I didn't want to fall asleep in here and have our daughter find us in bed together in the morning. I don't want to confuse her."

"Fine," he says stiffly.

He walks over to where his clothes are. He gets his boxer shorts and puts them on.

Then, he walks out of the room.

I put the rest of my clothes on and leave his bedroom.

I find him standing in the living room in the semi-darkness. His back to me, he stares out the window. I see the bottle of beer I got for him earlier dangling from his fingers.

"Zeus . . ." I say, feeling like I need to say something, but I'm cut off before I can say any more.

"Good night, Cameron."

His tone brokers no conversation, and honestly, it's a relief because I didn't actually know what I was going to say to him. I was just going to wing it.

I walk away and go into my and Gigi's room, quietly closing the door behind me. I don't even bother brushing my teeth. I just undress and pull on a clean nightshirt. Then, I climb in bed beside my baby girl, who has star-fished out in bed, taking up most of the room. Nothing new there.

I lie on my back and stare up at the darkened ceiling, wishing for answers that just won't come.

It's clear that I can't stay away from Zeus.

But I can't be with him either.

A silent tear of frustration runs down my cheek. I brush it away with my hand.

I'm such a mess.

And I fear that I'm just going to keep messing things up further. Because, when it comes to Zeus, I have zero control. And zero sense.

The man is my weakness. My downfall. My ruin.

He always has been.

And it seems that he always will be.

Chapter Twenty-Seven

Gigi's sleeping. Aunt Elle is downstairs, going over some case files. And I'm lying on my bed with my earbuds in, listening to music on my phone. Currently, P!nk is in my ears, telling me I need to "Try."

Maybe I do. Try to get Zeus out of my head and heart.

The asshole.

We got back from Disney World yesterday. And things have been difficult between us since we slept together that night.

Not so much that Gigi has noticed. But I've definitely noticed.

Clipped responses. Looking right through me like I barely exist.

It's not . . . nice.

Truthfully, it's annoying the crap out of me. He knew it was just sex. I'd told him that. He'd even repeated it back to me, for God's sake!

Yet he's pissed that I, what? Didn't cuddle after sex?

Because that wouldn't have given him the wrong idea, would it?

Ugh. I'm angry with him for being angry with me. He has no right. I've done nothing wrong.

Right?

So . . . why do I feel guilty? Why do I feel like the shittiest human being on the planet right now? And why is it annoying me so much that he's ignoring me?

Because you love him, you idiot.

If I'm being honest . . . the thing that's bothering me most is what happened when he was here earlier . . . well, more like what I saw.

Zeus was upstairs putting Gigi to bed and reading her a story, like usual.

I was tidying away Gigi's shoes that she'd left scattered all over the hall.

Zeus's cell was on the hall table, next to his car keys. I wasn't snooping, but his phone started ringing. I glanced at the screen and the display said, *Mindi Calling.*

Not gonna lie. I felt a stab of jealousy, knowing some woman was calling him.

I quickly brushed it off because she could be anyone. A friend. Someone who works in the boxing industry.

Then, his phone beeped a text a minute later.

I'm in NY for a few days. You wanna get together? It's been too long since I've had you inside me. ;)

Yep. No mistaking that.

He got a sext. While he was upstairs, reading a bedtime story to our daughter.

Mr. I Want You Back is sexting with this Mindi chick, and I want to stab myself in the eye with a blunt instrument. And throw up.

Screw him.

I didn't say anything to him when he came downstairs. Of course, he didn't say anything to me.

Just picked his cell and car keys up and left without giving me a backward glance.

Probably going to ring Mindi and meet for sex.

Mothereffing asshole.

I Googled his name along with Mindi's, and I got some hits.

Mindi Warrington is a pretty blonde pro tennis player that Zeus has been linked to on occasion. The last news story on them was five months ago, according to the date on the entertainment website. They were spotted entering a hotel together.

My cell phone screen nearly cracked, as I was pressing down on it that hard while reading.

I hate him. And her.

Well, I don't hate her. It's not her fault that Zeus is a gigantic ass. Who came here and invaded my life. Turned everything upside down. Promising me the earth. All the while, he's been sexting with Mindi, the perky tennis player.

Screw him.

Asshole.

He doesn't get to treat me like this. He doesn't get to come here with his insincere declarations, making promises of forever, while he's got another woman on the burner.

Ugh. I hate that he's turned me into a psychoanalyzing nutjob.

I yank my earbuds out and jump off my bed. I start pacing my room. Anger is pulsing through me.

I'm sick of him messing my life up.

I want him gone.

He can see Gigi. But *I* don't want to see him ever again.

We can set up an arrangement where he sees Gigi without me having to see his face. Maybe then, I'll finally be able to get over him.

Yeah, good luck with that.

No, I can do this. I'm gonna go and see him to tell him exactly how it's going to be.

I pocket my cell and leave my room. I look in on Gigi. Fast asleep.

I jog downstairs. I find Aunt Elle at the dining table, case files spread out on it.

"Hey, I need to go out for just a short while. You okay to watch Gigi? She's sleeping, so she won't bother you while you work."

She looks up from her reading, smiling. "Of course I am. And Gigi could never bother me. You know that." Her eyes focus in on my face and line with concern. "You okay?"

I realize that I'm tapping my foot with restless energy. I stop. "Yeah . . . I just need to talk to Zeus."

She nods but doesn't say anything, and I appreciate that.

"I won't be long."

"Take as long as you need."

I grab my car keys and leave the house.

On the short drive to Zeus's, Little Mix's "Nobody Like You" plays in my car, the words pricking at my heart.

I pull up outside his apartment. Get out of my car and walk the short distance to his door.

Reaching it, I ring the bell. Then, my brain decides to work.

What if he's not here? Or worse . . . what if Mindi's here?

Shit. I really didn't think this through.

God, I can be irrational at times.

I need to get out of here.

I step back to leave when the door opens, and he's standing there, wearing dark gray trackpants slung low on his hips and a fitted black T-shirt. His hair is damp, like he just had a shower.

What if he just got out of the shower because he got all sweated up from having sex with Mindi?

"Hi," he says.

I note a hint of caution in his tone, and pain leaks into my chest. My hands clench up into fists, nails biting into my skin.

"Are you alone?" I blurt out.

His brows come together. "Currently? Or in life?"

"Funny. I mean, do you have someone in your apartment right now?" *Specifically, in your bedroom.*

Eyes holding mine, he slowly shakes his head. "Nope. Just me here."

"You sure?"

He glances over his shoulder before looking back at me. "Yep. You wanna check?" He steps aside, widening the door.

"No."

"You sure?"

"Yep."

There's a beat of silence. Then, another.

"Did you come here to just check if I was alone?"

"No." *Kinda.* I brace myself, spine straightened, arms by my sides. "I came to tell you that I don't want to see you anymore. Of course, I would never stop you from seeing Gigi. But I can't be around you anymore. It's not good for me. *You're* not good for me. So, we need to figure something out regarding Gigi, whether it be Aunt Elle is there when you collect her or . . . I don't know. But we need to figure out something because I don't want to see you anymore."

"Says the woman standing on my doorstep."

"I came to tell you this." I frown.

"You could have called me."

True.

"Yeah, well, I'm not you. I don't do my dumping over the phone."

It's his turn to frown. "I didn't know we were together for you to dump me."

"Look"—I hold a hand up, stopping us before we start—"I didn't come here to verbally spar with you. I just came to tell you that we need to make other arrangements, so I don't have to see you every day."

I hear the chatter of people nearby, and I glance over my shoulder, but I don't see anybody.

"Come inside," Zeus tells me.

I don't argue because I don't want our business to be public knowledge.

I walk into his living room and stop by a wooden cabinet that has some of his boxing trophies on it. I turn around to face Zeus, who's standing across the room from me. I lean my ass against the cabinet and wrap my arms over my chest.

"So, what do you say?" I ask.

"No." He folds his arms over his huge chest, mirroring me.

"No?" I echo.

"That's not going to work for me," he says.

"What?" I blink.

He drops his arms and walks closer to me, lids lowering over his darkening eyes. "I said, that's not going to work for me."

"Well, this isn't about you and what works for you!" I throw my arms up in the air. "It's about me! And, I thought you'd be happy that we wouldn't have to see each other. You've been ignoring me since Disney World."

"I didn't handle it well. I was hurt. And I guess I thought that maybe, if I cold-shouldered you for a few days, it might make you realize a few things."

"Like?"

"Like . . . you still love me. That you want to be with me."

I realized that days ago. That's not the problem.

"You were playing games?"

He shakes his head, his eyes never leaving mine. "Fighting for you, Dove."

"Yeah, well, why don't you save your energy and stop fighting for me and go see Mindi, your perky tennis player? You won't have to fight at all for her, if her text was anything to go by."

Fucking fuck. Me and my big mouth.

"You read my text?" He doesn't seem angry. More like amused.

And that annoys the hell out of me.

"I saw it by accident."

"Mmhmm." He's nodding. A smile playing on his gorgeous lips. Lips that I could quite happily punch right now.

I'm feeling irritated and jealous, and I want to hurt him.

"Have you had sex with her since you've been with me?"

His smile drops, anger diluting his features, and I keep going because I know I'm getting the desired effect. And, also, because I don't care right now.

"Because I want to know if I need to get tested, considering you and I have had sex without a condom—twice."

His jaw tightens. "I get physicals on the regular, including tests for any diseases or infections, but you already know that. And the last time I had sex before you was about five months ago, and I've been checked since then. I always used condoms on the rare occasions that I had sex with other women. You're the only person I've ever gone unprotected with. What about you?"

I rear back. "What about me?"

"Well, you were screwing Deputy Dick. Maybe you still are. Did you use condoms, or do I need to get myself tested?"

I've never hit anyone in my life. Never. But I want to hit him right now.

But I won't. Because that's not who I am.

But I am a bitch. And I will hurt him in other ways that I know I can. Rightly or wrongly.

Not taking my eyes off Zeus, I reach behind me and grab one of his boxing trophies. Then, I throw it at the wall to my left with all my might. I hear the crack as it hits the wall and then the thud as it drops to the floor.

"Feel better?" he asks without a shred of emotion.

"No," I snap.

"So, break them all." He lifts a shoulder, taking a step toward me. "Tear the whole fucking place up, if it'll make you feel better. Do whatever you need to, so we can get past this and move forward."

I let out a bitter sounding laugh. "You just don't get it, Zeus. There is no moving forward because I can't forgive you!"

The next thing I know, he's in front of me, grabbing my face in his hands. "There has to be because I love you so fucking much." The raw emotion in his eyes and voice tears at me. "I know you love me, Cam. I know I'm not alone in this. We're the real fucking deal. Our love is what most people spend a lifetime searching for and never find. Don't throw us away, please."

"I didn't throw us away," I whisper brokenly. "You did."

"Fuck, Cam." He presses his forehead to mine. "I'm sorry. I'm so fucking sorry. Just forgive me, please. Because I can't spend my life without you."

He's surrounding me. His scent, his heat, his emotion. I can barely breathe, let alone think straight.

I step out of his hold, needing space.

His hands drop to his sides. His head lowers. He looks beaten.

I wrap my arms around myself. "Did you text her back?" I whisper.

His eyes lift to mine. "Yes."

A sound of anguish escapes me.

"I told her that my circumstances had changed," he's quick to say. "I said that I couldn't see her anymore."

I resent the relief I feel. "Why?"

"Why do you think?"

I lift my palms up.

"Because I'm not available, Dove. I haven't been since I was seventeen years old."

A pained laugh escapes me. "Yet you had sex with her five months ago."

"You slept with Deputy Dick."

"Because you left me!" I yell.

And, around and around, we go.

Zeus drags his hand over his head and down to the back of his neck, and he sighs. "I was lonely," he says quietly. "I was trying to fill the void of you. Not that it ever worked. But that's all it ever was. All it ever could be. Because I could never get over you."

The longing and aching in his eyes is too much for me to bear.

I turn away and walk over to the now broken trophy. I crouch next to it, and pick it up, instantly realizing which trophy I broke.

His first ever boxing trophy.

God, I'm a terrible person.

"I'm sorry," I say, standing back up, holding the two pieces in my hands. The boxing glove has broken off. The boot is still attached to the base. "Do you have glue?" I ask. "I can try to fix it."

"It's fine."

"No, I should be able to fix it," I continue. I lift it up, turning it over to see if the glove will reattach.

Something flutters out of the boot, falling to the carpet. Ticket stubs. Putting the trophy down, I bend down and pick them up. It takes me a few moments to realize what they are. And, when I do, my eyes flash to Zeus's, which are carefully watching me.

"Are these . . ." My mouth feels like cotton is stuffed in it. I swallow roughly and try again. "Are these the ticket stubs from the Ferris wheel ride? The first one we went on together?"

He nods, not saying a word.

"I didn't know you'd kept these . . . all these years. Why?"

He walks over to me. "Because they signify the moment I fell in love." His hand lifts to my face, and he tucks my hair behind my ear. "That smart mouth and those long legs . . . I never stood a chance." He smiles gently. "I kept those tickets to always remind me of what I had in case I ever forgot."

"You did forget," I whisper, tears filling my eyes.

He shakes his head. "I never forgot, Dove. I just let other things get in the way. I won't make that mistake again. Now, tell me you love me. And that you forgive me. And that we're gonna make this work."

I want to say yes. Knowing that he kept those ticket stubs for all these years has loosened something inside me. But, still, the fear of giving myself over to him and getting hurt again holds me back.

"I just . . . I ca—"

"Don't say you can't." He presses his fingertips to my lips, silencing me. "Just . . . let me show you something first. Then . . . decide."

My eyes lower. "I don't know, Zeus."

"Please, Dove."

I look back into his pleading eyes. Eyes I've loved since I was fifteen. And I whisper, "Okay."

Chapter Twenty-Eight

WE'RE IN ZEUS'S CAR, driving to whatever it is that he wants me to see.

Lady Gaga's "The Edge of Glory" is playing on the radio, and I'm wondering if he remembers when he says quietly, "Our prom song."

I glance at him. His eyes meet mine in the dark.

"Yeah," I say softly.

Clichéd as it is, it was after my senior prom that we had sex for the first time.

We'd been together for two years. We'd done pretty much everything but the act itself. I was ready. It was him that always held back.

He wanted to wait until I was eighteen. I was a few months shy of my eighteenth birthday. I didn't want to wait. Most of my high school friends had lost their virginity at sixteen. I was dating the hottest guy in Coney Island . . . the world . . . and I was still a virgin.

Anyway, he took me to prom, and it was everything I could have hoped it would be. Then, after, Zeus surprised me with a room in a really nice hotel. He was making half-decent money from his fights by that point. It wasn't long after that when he went to the Olympics and came back with gold, and his career took off.

The beginning of our end.

So, yeah, I gave him my body that night. He'd already had my heart.

I never did quite get it back the same.

I break eye contact and look out the passenger window of his car. He's driving down a private road. A lake is on the right.

"Where are we going?" I ask.

He turns into a driveway, pulling to a stop outside a beautiful, big, old colonial-style house with a wraparound porch.

"We're here," he says, turning off the engine. He gets out of the car.

Confused, I follow him.

"Here, where?" I ask, shutting the car door.

He turns to face me. "Home."

"This is yours?"

"Ours."

"I'm sorry, what?" I step forward, closer, sure I must've heard him wrong.

"It's ours. Yours, mine, and Gigi's. I bought it."

Then, he turns and walks up the porch steps. He unlocks the door.

My body kicks into action, and I follow him into the house. I step into a wide hallway. Staircase in front. Doors off to the sides.

I shut the door behind me and lean against it. "What do you mean, it's mine, yours, and Gigi's?"

"I bought it for us. I don't really know how else to phrase it."

I blankly stare at him. "You bought us a house."

"You need to know I'm not going anywhere." He spreads his arms out. "I'm not going anywhere, Dove. I bought this house because I want to be where you and Gigi are. And I'm hoping that, one day, you both will come to live here with me."

I'm still staring at him. I think I've gone into shock. My heart is beating wildly. "I can't believe you did this."

"Believe it."

"It's too much."

"No." He steps close to me, wrapping his hands around my biceps. "It's what needed to be done. This is me showing you that I'm not leaving. I tried telling you, and it didn't work. So, all I've got left are actions. I'm here to stay. This house is ours. I want us to live here as a family. I want to put my daughter to bed every night and then climb into bed beside you."

It sounds like everything I used to want. And that's why I say, "I can't move in with you."

"Why not?"

"Because . . ." I'm faltering for a reason as to why not, so I state the obvious, "We're not together."

"Babe, we're together, even when we're not."

I open my mouth to argue, but nothing comes out because he's right. Even when I wasn't with him, when I was hating him, I was still his because I could never truly let him go. And it was the same for him.

"We have history, Dove. But we have a future together, too. And our future is in this house." His hands slide up my arms to cradle my face. "The moment I saw this place, I saw us. Do you remember how we used to talk about one day having a house near the water with a wraparound porch, filling it with our kids once we were done with our life in the city? You would dance, and I would fight. Then, when it was time, we'd both step away, move to a place just like this, and start a family. You'd open up a dance school, and I'd maybe open up a boxing gym." His thumb sweeps over my cheek. "I know it didn't go the way we'd planned. I know that was because of me. But we can still have it. Still have the life we talked about together, starting now."

"You'd give up boxing?"

He holds my eyes. "After the Dimitrov fight. Once I bank that money, I'm done."

I exhale. "Zeus, I don't want you to stop boxing. I don't want you to give your career up because you think that's what I want."

"I want to be here with you and Gigi, and . . . I don't feel the same about it like I used to. Before, I used to love the thrill of the fight. Of course, the money mattered. But, now . . . that's all it's about."

"But the problem between you and me isn't the boxing, Zeus."

"You think I don't know that? You don't trust me to stay. You think I'm going to walk out on you again and never come back."

My eyes lower. He forces them back up.

"I can't prove it to you unless you give me the chance to."

He's right. I know he's right.

But fear is a cruel thing. It strangles you. Cripples

you. Stops you from saying the words you wish you could say.

He must see my internal struggle because he slips his hands from my face. Running one down my arm, he takes hold of my hand.

"Let me show you around."

I go with him, and he takes me first to the living room that has a gorgeous antique fireplace, but the decor is dated, as is the kitchen. Zeus tells me that he got the house for a good price for those reasons. That it won't cost a lot to update it.

As he gives me the tour, I can see the three of us living here. And that thought terrifies me.

"There are four bedrooms," he tells me as we reach the upstairs. "Gigi will have her pick from three. I think she'll love the bedroom at the front, as it overlooks the lake, but this"—he leads me toward an open door—"is the master. It has its own bathroom and balcony."

I step into the room. It's big and airy. The wallpaper on the walls is faded and peeling. But it's still amazing.

Wordlessly, I walk over to the doors leading out onto the balcony.

I turn the key in the lock, open them, and step outside.

The view is stunning. It overlooks the back garden and woodland behind the home. It's private and secluded. A piece of heaven.

I feel Zeus come up behind me.

"What do you think?" he says softly, his breath whispering down my neck.

"I think it's perfect, but—"

"Don't." His hands on my shoulders, he turns me to face him. "Don't say what you think you should say, what your hurt and anger are telling you to say. Tell me what's in your heart."

You. Always you.

I blow out a shaky breath, tears pricking at my eyes.

"Do you still love me?" he asks gently.

I can see the fear in his eyes. Fear that I'll tell him no, turn him away again. *That's* what makes me finally tell him the truth.

"Yes," I whisper.

"Then, we can make this work."

"But—"

"No *buts*, Dove. I love you. And you love me. We'll make this work."

I close my eyes, trying to gather my thoughts. "But Gigi . . . I can't risk . . ." I open my eyes to look at him. "I don't want her to get attached to the idea of us in case it doesn't work out."

"So, we keep it between you and me for now. We won't tell Gigi that we're together until you feel ready."

"And what about this house?"

"It's not going anywhere. I can work on getting it ready for us. And, when you're ready to move in, you and Gigi, I'll be here, waiting."

Everything he's saying is wonderful and perfect. But I'm scared. My pulse is racing. My heart chasing it.

"Cam . . ."

I blink up at him. "I'm afraid," I confess.

Pain floods his eyes. "I hate that I did this to you." He squeezes his eyes shut and presses his lips to my forehead. "I'm so fucking sorry." He kisses my temple.

"I'll never hurt you again. I swear." A kiss to my cheek. "Just let me back in, and I promise to spend the rest of my life taking care of you and Gigi. Let me fix us."

"What if you can't?" My voice is shaky.

I don't realize I'm crying until he brushes my tears away with his thumbs.

"*Can't* isn't an option, babe. I will fix us. And you will trust me again."

I squeeze my eyes shut, thinking—not with my fearful mind, but with my heart. The one that's loved him for nine years.

"Okay," I whisper, opening my eyes.

"Okay?"

"I'm willing to try. You and me."

His face is filled with so much happiness right now that I can't stop myself from smiling.

"Really?"

"Really. But we take it slow, and Gigi isn't to know until we're absolutely sure that we're going to work out."

"We're gonna work, baby."

Then, he grabs my face and kisses me as surely as his words. It's hard not to feel his happiness and excitement even though I'm still worried, wishing that I felt the same level of assuredness that we will work out as he does.

"I fucking love you," he says over my lips.

"I love you, too," I tell him for the first time in a long time. It's scary to say but also a damn relief. It's been so long since I've been able to say those words to him.

He pulls back from me, staring into my eyes, his shining with emotion that clutches at my chest. "Say it again."

I swallow nervously and lick my lips. His eyes drop to them.

"I love you."

His eyes roam my face, like he's memorizing the moment. Like he's never heard me speak those words before.

I feel a drop of rain hit my cheek. Then, another. It starts to rain. A gentle shower. The air still warm.

His finger touches my cheek, tracing a raindrop down to my lips.

I'm trembling inside. Needing him to touch all of me. Kiss me.

His fingers slide into my hair. He tugs my head back. And seals his mouth over mine.

I kiss him back with fervor.

We take our time undressing each other. Hands touching every inch of skin. Like we've never done this before.

Each caress, each kiss, tender and unhurried. Like we have all the time in the world.

And I guess we do.

Zeus's thick fingers dip inside me, agonizingly slow, driving me crazy. Making me desperate for him until I'm panting and begging for him to give me what I want.

Him.

Always him.

He backs me up to the wall of the house. My naked back against the wooden panels of the house. My skin wet from the rain.

I shiver. Not because I'm cold. But because of the man pressed up against me. The man I've always loved. The man I can't seem to stop loving.

Zeus's hand slides under my slick, wet thigh, lifting it, opening me up to him. He dips down until he's eye-level with me and presses his hips against mine. I feel the head of his cock push at my entrance. My hips shift restlessly, needing him inside me more than I need air right now.

"I love you," he whispers.

His lips brush over mine. Once. Twice. He sucks the rain off my lower lip, and then his teeth sink in, biting me, at the same moment he pushes inside me, inch by thick inch, until he's all the way inside me.

My eyes close on a moan. I love the euphoric feeling of having him inside me again.

"Tell me you love me," he says roughly. "I want to hear you say it while I'm deep inside you."

And he is deep. So very deep. Under my skin. He always has been.

I open my eyes and stare into his heavy-lidded, lust-filled eyes. "I love you," I tell him, breathless with need for him.

He groans, his eyes closing. He kisses me again and starts to move inside me. His rain-soaked body slick against mine.

And Zeus makes love to me out here, on the balcony of the house he bought for us, while the rain continues to shower down.

Chapter Twenty-Nine

"WHAT IS IT WITH us and rain?" I laugh softly.

We're in the living room, lying together on the sofa that the previous owners left here, covered with a blanket that Zeus grabbed from the trunk of his car. And, yes, he ran out there naked, to get it. Let's hope the neighbors down the road didn't see. Our wet clothes are drying in front of the fire that I got going while he did his birthday suit dash. Neither of us was clever enough to put our clothes inside to stop them from getting wet while we got busy on the balcony in the rain. Guess we were too caught up in the moment. Too caught up in each other.

"Well, I do love you wet." He turns his face to mine, grinning in that sexy way he does.

"Perv."

"Truthful," he counters.

I roll my eyes and shake my head, fighting to keep the smile off my face.

I'm feeling happy. It's been a long time since I felt

this kind of happiness. The happiness I've only ever been able to feel with him.

"All of our important moments in life seem to happen in the rain," I muse more to myself than him.

He starts to sing off-key, the words to Rihanna's "Umbrella."

Our song.

"Dork." I nudge him with my elbow, but secretly love that he remembers the song's importance.

He rolls onto his side, facing me, propping his head up with his hand. The flicker of flames glowing on his face. "I've missed that sound."

"What sound?"

"You laughing. Do it again."

"I can't laugh on command."

"I can make you."

"So, do it," I challenge, raising my brow. "Just don't sing again."

"Funny."

There's a brief pause.

Then, he attacks, and he knows exactly where to go—my stomach. I'm ridiculously ticklish.

"Ah! Stop!" I laugh, trying to bat his hands away but to no avail.

"No, I haven't heard enough."

"Zeus!" I scream with laughter, my chest aching in the best possible way. "Come on! Stop!"

"Okay," he grumbles, relinquishing his tickle assault on me. He flops onto his back.

"I really fucking missed you," he says quietly, turning his suddenly serious eyes to mine.

I press my hand to his chest, over his heart, touching my tattoo. "I missed you, too," I tell him. I dip my head and kiss him.

As I pull back, his hand comes into my hair, holding me there. "I know I screwed up with us. I won't make that mistake again."

"I know," I whisper.

But we both know I only half-believe that. I'm not fully in that place where I believe him yet.

He pulls me back down to his lips and languidly kisses me.

I lay my head down on his chest, tangling my legs with his.

The sound of the fire crackling in the background and the beat of his heart in my ear—this is all I need right now.

"Do you remember when you performed at the winter showcase to 'Umbrella'?" he says out of nowhere.

"Of course I remember." I roll my eyes. The piece I choreographed was about him and me, about how I felt about him from the moment I'd met him. How I've always felt about him. "Where did that come from?" I ask him, tipping my head back to look into his eyes.

He lifts a shoulder. "I don't know. I remember everything about us . . . but it's just one of those memories that has always stuck with me. Watching you dance was my favorite thing in the whole world. I hate that you don't dance anymore."

"I was dancing—at the club." Until I quit when he made a reappearance in my life.

"You know that's not what I meant." His eyes darken. "I hate that you stopped because of me."

"I stopped because I was pregnant. If you'd been there or not, I still would have had to drop out."

"But you could have gone back if I'd been there to support you."

I shake my head. "I wouldn't have gone back. What would have been the point? I had Gigi, and she was the most important thing to me. You know how ballet is. It's grueling, long hours. I wasn't going to spend that kind of time away from her."

His eyes go to the ceiling. He blows out a hard breath. "Still, I should've been there."

I don't say anything. Because he's right. He should've been there. I can blame Marcel for Zeus not being there for Gigi. But not for Zeus not being there for me. He's to blame for that.

His eyes, determined and steady, come back to mine. "I will make it up to you both. I swear to you, Dove."

I slide my hand up to his face, pressing my palm to his cheek. "You already are by just being here right now."

But I know the look in his eyes. I know he thinks he should be doing more. Hence, the purchase of this house.

"Zeus . . . you didn't have to buy this house, you know."

I know he's okay for money, but he's still putting Lo and Missy through college and financially supporting his dad. He has money, but that money will also have to last him when his boxing career does finally come to an end.

His brows draw together. "Yes, I did. You need to know that I'm here to stay. And I will do whatever it takes to show you that."

"I just . . . I know you have money. I just don't want you wasting it."

Frustration lines his eyes. "Nothing spent on you or Gigi is a waste. And I'm good for money, Cam. Don't worry about that."

"So, why is the Dimitrov fight so important? You said to me a while ago that you were doing it because you needed the money."

He looks away from me. Too quickly. "I need to secure Gigi's future."

I believe that. I do. But I also think there's something else he's not telling me. Some other reason he needs the money.

I'm about to probe when he says, "Will you dance for me?" He brings his eyes back to mine. They're thoughtful and clear. Whatever was bothering him a moment ago has gone.

"Now?"

"Yeah."

"Er . . . no." I laugh.

"Why not?" His lips frown at me.

"Because I'm naked." I wave a hand down myself.

"And?" He raises a brow.

"And I'm not dancing naked."

"Strippers do."

"I'm not a stripper, you big jerk!"

I gently jab him in the chest, and he laughs. Catching my hand, he brings it to his lips and brushes a kiss over my knuckles.

"No, you're not. You're my very limber ballerina."

His big hand slides down my thigh, lifting it up his

body, making me shiver when he palms my ass and squeezes.

I want him again. And the hardness beneath my leg is telling me that he wants me again, too.

But I'm also conscious of the time. I've been out for much longer than I first anticipated already. I know Aunt Elle is home, and she doesn't mind. But I mind.

And, no matter how much I want to stay here in this bubble with him and stretch out our time together, I have a little girl waiting for me at home.

"Do you think our clothes are dry by now?" I ask him. "I should really get home."

Zeus's wanting expression quickly changes into one of disappointment.

"I reckon so," he says, sounding despondent.

"Hey . . ." I touch my fingers to his chin. "I don't want to go. But I've been out for way too long already. It's not fair for Aunt Elle," I say gently.

"You don't have to explain yourself. You need to get home to our daughter. I get it."

"But?"

His eyes flash at me. "There's no *but*."

"There was definitely a *but*," I challenge.

He sighs and looks up at the ceiling again. "It's stupid."

"Nothing you have to say is stupid."

There's a sizable pause, before he says in a low voice, "I'm worried."

I cup his cheek and draw his eyes back to mine. "About?"

Another breath. "That you're going to leave here . . . me . . . go home, and change your mind about us."

I stroke my thumb over the scar on his brow. "I'm not going to change my mind."

"I just . . . can't be without you again," he whispers, sounding vulnerable.

It tugs at my chest, making me ache for him.

I can't recall the last time I heard Zeus sound this way. He's always so sure of himself and others. Even when I was fighting against us being together, he was telling me that it was inevitable. And he was right.

I thought I was the only one with fears over losing him again.

But it's clear he's worried about losing me, too.

Zeus might have been the one to leave me all those years ago, but that doesn't mean any of it was easy on him. It's clearly left scars on him, too. And, somehow, that makes me feel less alone . . . less fearful of doing this with him.

"So, don't be without me," I say softly.

His hands come around my face, thumbs spanning my cheeks, as he stares into my eyes. "Babe, the only thing that could take me away from you is death. And I don't plan on dying anytime soon. It's not me I'm worried about. It's you. I'm scared that you're going to see sense and shut me out again."

Scared.

Zeus Kincaid is scared. His whole persona revolves around him being fearless. Yet here he is, telling me that he's afraid I'm going to leave him.

"I've never heard you say that you're afraid."

He lets out a self-deprecating laugh. His eyes stay

steady on mine. "*You* fucking terrify me, Dove. You always have. The way I feel about you . . ."

Something inside me cracks wide open at his admission. "You terrify me, too," I admit quietly. "My feelings for you. And you don't have to worry about me seeing sense and leaving you because, clearly, I've never had any sense when it comes to you." I grin to add levity to the seriousness of the moment.

His lips lift into that smile of his, the one that can heal and break my heart, all at the same time.

"Glad to hear it," he says before kissing me one last time. "Now, come on." He pats my ass with his hand. "Let's check on these clothes to make sure they're dry and get you home to our girl."

Chapter Thirty

IT'S EARLY. I BARELY slept a wink last night, and this time, I wasn't awake with uncertainty over my decision to be with Zeus. Okay, there might have been a little bit of uncertainty, but mostly, there was smiling and heart flips every time I thought of last night with him. I must have run every single moment of the night over in my head about a hundred times.

Every word he'd spoken to me, every touch, every kiss. Every second of the way he'd made love to me. Like it was our first time.

God, I feel like a teenager again. Reminiscent of how I felt when we first started dating.

Only I'm older and wiser this time. Hence, the caution accompanying the fluttery, floating-on-a-cloud feelings.

I'm staring out the kitchen window, my hands wrapped around my coffee cup, when Aunt Elle wanders into the kitchen, still dressed in her pajamas.

"Hey, couldn't sleep?" she comments at my being up early.

"No," I say. But I smile, so she knows not to be concerned. There's usually something wrong if I'm out of bed early.

"Gigi still in bed?" she asks, pouring a coffee.

"Yeah. I looked in on her before I came down, and she was still out for the count."

Aunt Elle chuckles. "Like mother, like daughter."

I flash a smile at her. "I'll get her up soon."

We need to start getting ready for the day. I have work, and Gigi has pre-K.

"So, how did things go with Zeus last night? You got back late."

"Sorry." My cheeks flush like a guilty teenager.

"Don't apologize. You're a grown woman."

"And a mother."

"I was here all night, Cam. It doesn't matter what time you came home. I just want to make sure everything is okay with you."

I can't keep the smile off my face. I bring my cup to my lips, trying to cover it.

But she sees. And she grins. "So, from that smile, should I take it that everything is good between you and Zeus?"

I take a sip of coffee and hold the cup to my chest.

"He bought a house." Pause. "For him . . . me, and Gigi."

Her eyes widen. "Wow."

"Yeah." I sigh. "He says he's here to stay, and he wants me to know that. Also, he wants us to live with him."

"Okay. And what did you say?"

I bite my lip.

Aunt Elle has never judged my choices, and she's

never made comments on any of the decisions I've made in my life, especially since Zeus has come back. But I still feel worried over what she might think of us getting back together. After everything that happened between Zeus and me, she was there with me at my lowest points. After he left, she saw how wrecked I was, and then she had to witness the devastation I went through when I believed he wanted nothing to do with our baby. I'm concerned that she'll think I'm nuts to give him another chance and risk getting hurt again.

Although she did collude with him behind my back on the Disney World trip, so maybe she won't be as opposed to the idea as I think she might be.

"I said no to living with him, of course. But I did say . . ." I pause again, biting the inside of my lip. Then, I blow out a breath and tell her, "I said I'd give him another chance. So, I guess we're back together. But we're taking it slow." I'm quick to say, "And we're not telling Gigi until I know for sure that I can trust him again and make it work."

She doesn't say anything. Just nods her head and takes a sip of her coffee. I can feel myself starting to crack.

"You think I'm crazy for giving him another chance, don't you?"

"Are you happy?" she asks me out of left field.

I don't have to think about this because I know the answer. "Yes."

"Then, that's all I care about. You're smart. You always have been. You don't make decisions lightly. I know you thought this through in a hundred different ways before deciding to give him another chance. And, no matter how much I would love to kick his ass for hurting you all those years ago, I also know from what you told me that he had his reasons. Right or wrong, he did what he thought he had to. He hurts you again, and I'll bury him." She grins, making me laugh. "But he loves you. I see the way he looks at you, same way he's always looked at you—like you're his entire world. And he's a great father to Gigi. So, to answer your question, no, I don't think you're crazy."

"That was quite a speech." I grin, the unease I felt before quickly ebbing away.

"I know. I impress myself with my awesomeness at times." She flashes a smile at me. "You want some breakfast?"

I don't get a chance to respond to her question as my cell phone starts to ring on the counter, interrupting us.

"It's Zeus," I say, seeing his name on the display. Butterflies swoop from my stomach and up into my chest, making me feel giddy.

I'm ridiculous. I've known Zeus forever. We have a child together. It's not like this is a new relationship. Still, it somehow feels new.

Aunt Elle gives me a knowing smile and heads for the door, coffee in hand. "I'll leave you to it."

"Hey," I answer on a smile. "I haven't changed my mind about us, if that's what you're calling to check on."

There's a brief pause.

Then, he says, "I'm outside. Can you come to the door?"

"My door?" I say stupidly.

"Yeah. I . . . need to talk to you."

Well, if that doesn't make me nervous, nothing will.

"Okay. I'm coming."

I hang up my cell, slipping it into the pocket of my pajamas. I walk quickly and quietly to the front door, my stomach churning with nerves. A hundred scenarios as to why he's here at this time in the morning are flashing through my mind. The main thought being that he's here to tell me he's leaving, which is stupid. I know he loves me and is here to stay.

He said that before, remember? the scared voice in my head reminds me.

I unlock the door and open it.

Zeus is standing on the porch, close to the steps. He's wearing running shorts and a tank. His skin is covered in a fine sheen of sweat.

He doesn't make a move to come over, and that has me even more worried.

"You want to come in?" I ask.

He shakes his head.

He doesn't want to come in. That's not a good sign.

I step out onto the porch and shut the door behind me. The wood is cold beneath my bare feet. I wrap my arms around myself, warding off the chill I feel.

"You ran here?" I ask, referring to his clothes.

"Yeah. I needed to burn off some energy."

His eyes quickly move off me. Like he's afraid to look at me. That means he's keeping something from me. And he's restlessly moving his hands, clenching his fists in and out, which means he's agitated. Those have always been his tells. In this moment, I hate that I know him so well.

"What's going on?" I curse the tremor in my voice.

The sound of me speaking brings his eyes back to

mine. I expect them to be closed off, like they always are when he doesn't want me to know what's going on with him.

But, instead of shuttered eyes, I see them shimmering with unease.

Dropping my arms to my sides, I take a step closer to him. "Zeus, what's going on?" I say more forcefully. "You're starting to scare me."

"Shit. Sorry." He steps forward and then stops before reaching me. He pushes his fingers through his hair and blows out a breath. "There's something I need to tell you."

Oh God. Here we go.

"It's not about me and you," he's quick to say. "Well, it is about me and you. But not in the way you think."

"I don't know what to think right now because you're not making much sense." I pull my pajama sleeves over my hands, holding on to the fabric with my fingers.

"Sorry. I just . . . fuck." He fixes his eyes on me. "My publicist called me last night while you and I were together. But I had my phone turned off. After I dropped you home, I turned it back on and saw that I had a bunch of missed calls and messages from him."

"What did he want? And what does this have to do with me?"

"Before I tell you, you need to know that I've been up all night, trying to fix this. To stop it from happening, but . . . it was too late."

"Fix what, Zeus?" My voice is firmer now because I want to know what the hell is going on. My heart hasn't pounded this hard with fear since the night he broke up with me over the phone.

"A story went out last night on Pharos."

It's one of those trashy news sites, which I'm ashamed to admit that I peruse from time to time.

"About . . . well, you."

"Me?" My hand goes to my chest in shock. "Why would there be a story about me on there?"

"The pictures of us together in Disney World. I guess they piqued some piece-of-trash journalist's interest. It makes sense because, as far as anyone knows, I'm a single guy. And then I'm there at Disney with you and Gigi. I should have considered this before I took you both there, but I don't pay much attention to the press, except for when I have to for fights."

"What are they saying? You said the story is about me, right? So, what's been said? That we have a child together? You and I are together? What?"

His eyes do a tour of everything but me, and my stomach drops through the floor because I know I'm not going to like what he's about to say.

His eyes meet mine again. "They're saying you got pregnant and didn't tell me. That you kept Gigi from me. That you work at a police station during the day, and at night, you . . ."

"What?" I demand.

"Strip. They're saying you work as a stripper."

Chapter Thirty-One

"I DO WHAT?" THE WORD bellows from my lungs, actually forcing myself back a step. "A stripper? A fricking stripper? They said I'm a stripper? I'm *not* a stripper! I was a go-go dancer! Not once have I taken my clothes off for money! Not that there's anything wrong with that, but I haven't done it! And I most definitely didn't keep Gigi from you!"

He comes to me. His big hands wrapping around my biceps. "I know that, Dove. But some asshole made up this bullshit story and printed it."

"Well, that's just fucking great!" I pull from his hold, moving away, needing some space. I walk to the edge of the porch and curl my hands around the railing, taking in and exhaling a few breaths. I tilt my head in his direction. "Can they do this? Print lies like this?"

I almost want to slap myself in the face for asking that. *Of course they can. The press is notorious for printing whatever they damn well feel like, truth or not.*

"I'm sorry," he says, sounding remorseful.

"Why are you sorry?" I straighten up, facing him,

one hand still holding on to that railing. It's like I need the support to ground me, so I don't run from here and straight to the person who printed this crap about me to kick the bullshit right out of them. "It's not like you printed these lies about me. It's not your fault this is happening."

He lets out a self-deprecating noise through his nose. "Babe, everything that goes wrong in your life is because of me. This is no exception. They wouldn't have targeted you if I were just some normal guy. It's because of what I do for a living . . . who I am to them. It makes me newsworthy. Meaning they will spin whatever shit they can to make a story sound juicer."

"God, it makes me so angry!" I rage, teeth gritted. "I can't believe they just get to do this! And, now, people are going to think I'm a stripper. What if the kids at school say mean stuff to Gigi? And—" My thoughts are spiraling out of control.

"It's going to be all right, Cam."

"No, it's not!" I yell at him. But I'm not yelling at him; I'm yelling at the asshole who printed this story. "It's not your name that's currently getting tarnished. It's mine!" I bang a hand to my chest, tears trying to force their way up.

I grab my cell from my pajama pocket and pull up a search engine. I type my name in it.

"What are you doing?" Zeus steps closer.

"Finding out exactly what people are saying about me."

"That's not a good idea."

He goes to wrap his hand over my phone, but I move it out of the way.

"I have to know."

My page fills with news stories, the headlines screaming at me.

Zeus Kincaid Has a Secret Child!
Click here to read all about his
secret daughter and the stripper who
kept his baby from him.

Zeus Kincaid and the Stripper Who
Had His Baby and Kept It Secret For
Four Years—Until Now. Click here
for the full exposé.

Everything You Need to Know About
Cameron Reed, Stripper and Zeus
Kincaid's Baby Mama. Click here to
read more.

I click on the third link. The page loads, and the first thing I see is a picture of me—a seriously unflattering picture of me dancing on a podium at the club. There's a pole, and I'm holding on to it, head thrown back, leg curled around it. I'm wearing sparkly hot pants and a matching bra top. I look like I could be pole-dancing. Or stripping.

"Jesus . . ." I groan, staring at the picture, unable to look away.

Zeus slides my phone from my hand and from my view, and I let him. "You don't need to see those."

"I never stripped." I look up at him with imploring eyes, knowing how incriminating that picture looks.

"I know that. But, even if you had, it wouldn't have mattered. What you do is no one's business but yours."

"I know. But . . . I just wanted to keep dancing, and it was fun. If I'd known . . . I never would have taken the job. Fuck!" I cry out.

He takes my face in his hands, staring into my eyes. "And, if you'd never taken that job, I wouldn't have seen you that night. I wouldn't have known about Gigi. And we wouldn't be together right now."

The front door flies open. Zeus releases me, turning to the door. Probably thinking the same as me—that it's Gigi. But it's not. It's Aunt Elle.

"What the hell is going on out here?" she hisses. "I could hear you yelling from upstairs. FYI, you woke up Gigi. You've about six seconds before she's down here."

"Fuck," I whisper. I press my hand to my forehead, turning to Aunt Elle. "The press has put out a story about me. They're saying I'm a stripper and that I didn't tell Zeus about Gigi. Jesus, they're painting me out to be a terrible mother." Angry tears fill my eyes.

I honestly don't think I've ever seen Aunt Elle look as livid as she does right now. Her eyes flick to Zeus.

"What are you doing about this? You have people, right? Can they put a stop to this?"

"I spent all night trying to put a stop to it. My publicist is still on it now, and my lawyer is talking to their lawyers. But I don't know what good it'll do. Pharos says they've got credible info and story corroboration from people who know Cam well."

"Bullshit," Aunt Elle says, sounding as dismayed as I feel.

"People like who?" I say. "No one knows about our history, about you not knowing about Gigi until recently. Well, apart from the three of us standing here. And Ares, Lo, and Missy."

"Who would never talk to the press," Zeus affirms.

I nod in agreement.

"Your dad?" I say, hating to say it, but it has to be said.

"He's too drunk to know the time of day. He barely remembers he has kids, let alone a granddaughter. So, that leaves . . ."

"Well, Rich knows, but—"

"Deputy Dick? You talked to that prick about us?"

"He's my friend."

"Who you used to fuck."

"Zeus . . ." I warn. "I trust Rich, and I know he wouldn't do something like talk to the press. I mean, come on. He's in law enforcement, for God's sake."

"And that means what?"

"That he knows not to talk to the press."

The derogatory laugh he lets out has me grinding my teeth and feeling surprised that Aunt Elle hasn't said anything.

"I can't believe you're defending that prick," he growls at me.

"I'm not!" I throw my hands up, frustrated. "I just know he wouldn't do that. What about Marcel? He just loves to talk to the press."

That asshole loves the sound of his own voice.

"Why would he?"

"Why wouldn't he? He kept your daughter's existence from you. Why not smear my reputation while he's at it?"

"Marcel doesn't know that I know about Gigi."

"You haven't confronted him about it yet? Why the hell not? Are you afraid of him?"

His eyes lift upward, and he lets out a disbelieving laugh. "Yeah, that's it, Cam. I'm afraid to talk to Marcel. I could kill the guy with one punch, but yeah, I'm terrified of him."

"So, why not say something to him?"

"Because I'm trying to be smart about it for once. It's not that I'm not doing anything because I am. Behind the scenes, I'm doing things, going for the guy where it's going to really hurt him, but it'll take time. But I know, if I go see Marcel anytime soon, I'll be spending the next twenty-five to fifty in a state penitentiary for murder. And, as much as I hate to admit it, I'm contracted to the bastard for my next fight. So, right now, dodging prison and keeping my income are my top priorities now that I have you and Gigi to provide for!"

"I don't need your money!"

"And I don't give a fuck! It's yours anyway!"

"Okay, back to your corners, children." Aunt Elle stands between us, arms spread out. "I'm pretty sure the whole street just heard that. That means—"

"Mommy?" Gigi's tiny voice comes from the doorway, and my heart dies in my chest.

I whirl around to her, and the worried look on her face makes me want to find a time machine, go back in time, and tell myself to shut the fuck up.

"Hey, Gigi girl." I go over and scoop her up into my arms.

"Are you and Daddy fighting?"

"No," I lie. "We're just disagreeing. You know, like

when you and April Sinclair have a falling-out at pre-K."

April is Gigi's best friend, and they argue like sisters would.

"You means, when *Apwil* takes the toys I'm *pwaying* with, and it makes me angry."

"Yeah, kinda like that, baby."

"So, did Daddy takes something of yours?"

My heart. My virtue. Yep. He definitely took some things of mine and never gave them back.

"Not so much took something. We just disagreed on a subject."

Zeus comes up behind me, touching his large hand to my shoulder, and cups Gigi's tiny face in his other hand. "Mommy and Daddy got a little angry with each other, and we yelled. And we're sorry."

"Has you said sorrys to each other? 'Cause Miss Maple says we has to says sorry when we yells at each other."

Zeus's hand on my shoulder slides up to the side of my head, and he presses his lips to my hair. "I'm sorry, Dove. I shouldn't have lost my temper."

I turn my eyes to his. "I'm sorry, too."

"Yous can be best *fwiends* now," Gigi says like she's officiating, making me smile.

"But you're my best friend," I tell her, pretending to frown.

"Don'ts be silly. You's my mommy. You can't be my best friend." She giggles, and my heart is full again.

"Hey, Gigi girl." Aunt Elle comes over and takes her from my arms, carrying her. "You wanna help me make breakfast? I was thinking . . . waffles and bacon."

"And maple syrup?"

"And maple syrup," Aunt Elle agrees.

"You's da best, Granny Elle. We can make waffles and bacon for Mommy and Daddy, too."

"For sure, Gigi girl."

I watch them go inside. Leaving the front door open for us.

Zeus turns me to face him. I stare up into his eyes.

"I'm sorry," he says again. "I'm an asshole."

"Yeah, you are," I agree. "But so am I."

"No." He shakes his head. "You're just hurt and scared, and I handled it badly. I fucked up again."

Tears fill my eyes. He cradles my face in his hands.

"But I'll fix this, Dove. Whatever it takes. Whoever I have to take down. I'll do whatever is necessary to make this go away."

Chapter Thirty-Two

BUT IT DOESN'T GO away.

Not that Zeus didn't try. Because he did. Pharos took the story down the next day after Zeus threatened to sue. But it's no use because the story is on every other gossip site known to man.

He had his publicist put out a statement on his social media, stating the facts—but leaving out Marcel's involvement. I hate that the asshole is getting off easy, but Zeus assured me that he won't. He also can't publically put the blame on Marcel for keeping Zeus from us, not without a mess of a fight on his hands. And, with the fact that he's contracted to Marcel for the Dimitrov fight, it makes everything so much more difficult. So, the statement went out, saying that mitigating factors had played a part in Zeus not knowing about his daughter up until recently, but that I was in no way to blame. And, that I'm not a stripper. But the press wasn't interested. A few small media sports outlets posted his statement, but it's not juicy in the terms of what the media wanted, so it didn't make the big headlines, and it just fell into the rest of the slush pile.

Me being a stripper and terrible mother is way juicier.

Zeus thinks it's all his fault. He thinks, by not protecting me from this or being able to fix it, it somehow makes him a failure.

I've told him that he can't protect me from everything.

People might think he's a god. But he's not. He's human. He bleeds like the rest of us.

He isn't used to losing a fight though. So, this has been hard on him. And me, too.

I started to wonder if this was some kind of omen. We'd just gotten back together, and then this happened.

But Zeus quickly talked that thought out of my head.

Of course, the press came to town. I had photographers following me when I was taking Gigi to pre-K. The one good thing about working at the precinct is that they look after their own. Whether they think you're a stripper or not. I might not be an officer, but when you work at the precinct, you're as good as one.

So, Port Washington's law enforcement have made it very clear to the press that they're not welcome here.

It's been well over a week now, and the press seems to be losing interest, which is good news for me.

But, sadly, the other moms at pre-K don't seem to be losing interest, and I'm still the top story of the moment. I don't know if it's because of who Zeus is. Or that they think I'm a stripper. Or that they think I purposely kept Zeus from his daughter. Or all three. Either way, my patience is wearing thin.

No one's said anything directly to me yet, but I'm getting the stares and disapproving looks from the moms, along with leers from some of the dads, and I've been hearing the whispers about me when they think I'm not listening.

Zeus wanted to do school drop-off with me, so I wouldn't be alone, but I told him no. It's bad enough when he's not there. Could you imagine the looks I would get if he was?

I just don't want any unnecessary attention brought Gigi's way.

She's doing fine. Of course, she asked why people wanted to take our pictures. And I just told her it was because Daddy's a famous boxer, and she was satisfied with that. She even started waving at the photographers, and I didn't stop her.

I did speak to her pre-K teacher when the story first broke. Not the most comfortable of conversations, but I wanted her to be in the know. She was great. And, apparently, she's a big boxing fan. Meaning a big fan of Zeus's. Insert eye roll here.

And we had no problems at all—up until yesterday. Well, it wasn't so much a problem. More of a question when I buckled Gigi up in her car seat and started the drive home.

"Mommy, what's a stwipper?*"*

I had to stop myself from slamming on the brakes. And bursting into tears.

I kept myself together and continued driving the car. "Where did you hear that word, baby?" I asked her.

"Well, at recess, Bentley Parsons said to me that he heard his mom tell his dad that you's a stwipper.*"*

I felt my heart crack down the middle.

"Bentley said to you that Mommy is a stripper?"

"My mommy, not his. He said his mommy's a party pwanner. *What's a party* pwanner?*"*

"Someone who plans and organizes parties for other people." And, gossips about other people and gives their kid a stupid name.

"I thinks I wants to be a party pwanner *when I's a grown-up."*

"I think you'd be an excellent party planner, Gigi girl." I smiled at her in the rearview mirror.

It was quiet for a moment, and I thought I'd dodged a bullet—until she said, "You didn't answer my question, Mommy."

My heart sank. "What question was that?"

She sighed and rolled her eyes. "I said, what's a stwipper?*"*

I knew there was no avoiding it, and I wasn't going to lie to her, so I took a deep breath and told her the truth, "Well, a stripper is a person who dances in front of people as a job, like Mommy did at the club, but the difference is that a stripper removes their clothes, and Mommy never did that when she danced."

I glanced at her in my rearview again and saw that her eyes were as wide as saucers.

"They gets naked?" she whispered.

"No, not totally naked. They keep their underwear on."

Okay, so I had to lie a little. I didn't want to scar her little mind for life.

"So, Gigi, if Bentley Parsons or anyone else says that your mommy is a stripper, you tell them they're wrong."

"Oh, I dids, Mommy. I said he was a big, fat wiar. *I said that's my mommy is a ballerina, and she's the most beautiful ballerina ever."*

Then, I did cry. Not because I was sad. Well, a little because I was sad. But mostly because I had the best kid in the whole world.

Zeus has brought me out to dinner. He said we needed to get out and spend some time together. Aunt Elle offered to look after Gigi. They're having pamper and movie night.

We've come to Louie's Oyster Bar & Grille. They do amazing seafood, and we're seated at a table that offers both privacy and a great view over Manhasset Bay.

But it seems that privacy still isn't enough. Because not long after we've placed our order for food, someone having dinner there gets up from their table and comes over to ask for Zeus's autograph. And that brings more people.

Zeus obliges, signing autographs and even posing for a few pictures.

I'm trying not to feel resentful. But, after having a camera shoved in my face for over a week, my patience is starting to wear thin.

I get that these people support him. But they could also be the people listening to the gossip being spread, and spreading it themselves.

"I'm going to the restroom," I tell Zeus, pushing my chair out, as he talks boxing with this overly eager thirty-something woman.

I take my time in there. Reapplying my lipstick, fluffing

out my hair. I'm basically wasting time before I have to go back to our dinner for two, plus one and whoever else might have turned up.

I exit the restroom, and I'm surprised to see Zeus leaning against the opposite wall, waiting for me.

"You okay?" he asks.

I nod.

"Let me ask again. Are you okay? And don't lie this time."

I narrow my eyes at him. "No," I answer truthfully. "We've had a shitty week. And we're supposed to be here, spending time together, but the only time we've actually done that tonight was in the car on the way here because since we arrived, everyone else has been commanding your attention. And I know that it's not your fault. But I'm feeling pissy and irrational right now, so I'm blaming you."

"So . . . am I to take it that you're not enjoying yourself?"

My eyes flash to his, and the fucker is smiling.

"Ass." I give him a shove in his shoulder.

He grabs hold of my wrist and hauls me into his big body, wrapping his arms around me. He brushes his lips over me, and I relax at his touch . . . his taste.

"I'm sorry," he says, pressing his forehead to mine. "I wanted tonight to be just ours, too."

I sigh. "I know. It just sucks at the moment."

"You wanna get out of here? Go somewhere that sucks a little less?"

"Or sucks better," I quip.

He chuckles deep. I feel the vibrations from his chest creep into mine.

I tip my head back a little and stare into his eyes. "We've already ordered our food," I say grimly.

"They're wrapping the food up as we speak, so we can take it with us."

My brow lifts. "So, we were already leaving?"

He gives me a boyish smile. "I know you well, Dove."

"Clearly."

He presses his lips to mine again. "I was thinking we could take the food back to my place, and I could use you as my dinner plate."

"This is a fish restaurant."

I wrinkle up my nose, and he laughs.

"I'm sure there's a bad sex joke in there somewhere," he says.

I playfully frown at him.

"Okay, so no eating food off your body." He puts his lips to my ear, making me shiver. "I guess I'll just have to eat you instead." He slips his hand between our bodies and cups me through my dress, pressing his fingers into me.

I moan softly, and he kisses me again, sinking his teeth into my lower lip, tugging on it.

"Let's go," he growls.

Chapter Thirty-Three

Zeus leads me back out into the restaurant. Our food is ready to go at the counter. As Zeus already paid, we're out of there and heading for his car. His arm is around me, and I'm staring into his face, listening to the dirty things he's whispering about, including what he's going to do to me when he gets me home.

We're so wrapped up in each other that we don't see him at first. It's the sound of the camera snapping pictures that captures my attention. I've been hearing that sound for over a week now, so I'm well accustomed to it.

And I've gotten familiar with the paparazzi hanging around, taking pictures. But this guy . . . I don't know.

"Ignore him," Zeus says, drawing me closer to his body as he walks us to his car.

"Hey, Zeus! How do you feel about your baby mama keeping your daughter from you? You seem okay by the looks of things. So, you guys are back together? Does that mean you're giving up stripping, Cameron?"

My face is going beet red. I'm shaking. I just want to get out of here and away from this guy.

"Why did you strip, Cameron? For the money? Or do you just like taking your clothes off for people? You know, there are people who'd pay good money to see you naked. Me included."

Zeus whirls around, letting go of me. He steps up to the pap. "Back the fuck off," Zeus barks at him.

The pap holds his hands up and takes a step backward. "Just stating facts, man." He gives a shrug.

"No, you're talking shit," Zeus growls.

I slide my trembling hand into Zeus's and tug on it. "Let's just go, Zeus. Please."

Zeus's eyes come to mine. Angry and frustrated. It feels like for ever before he nods his agreement, and then we're moving again. Quicker this time.

Zeus's car is mere feet away.

The pap is still following us though. I think the guy must have a death wish.

"Hey, Cameron, can you confirm whether the rumors that you also used to sleep with men for money are true?"

It happens so fast that I'm helpless to stop it.

The bag of food is thrown to the ground, and Zeus has the pap by the throat. His big hand around the guy's neck, he shoves the pap backward, practically lifting him off his feet, hitting his back into Zeus's car. His camera drops to the floor with a loud crack.

"Zeus!" I cry, my hands reaching for his arms, trying to pull him off the guy, who's gasping for air, his face reddening by the second.

But Zeus isn't letting go. It's like he doesn't even know I'm here right now.

"Say that again, motherfucker. To my face," Zeus grinds the words out through his clenched jaw.

"I-I didn't say anything," the pap chokes out.

Zeus leans his face into the guy's. "Liar. Say it."

"Zeus, let him go," I plead. "It doesn't matter what he said." I tug on the arm that has the guy by the throat. "Please. Think of Gigi."

The instant I say her name, I feel his muscles slacken in his arm, and I know I've reached him.

"Please, Zeus," I beg again.

His eyes turn to mine. The look in them . . . I've seen that look on him only one time outside of the ring, and it was when that guy was hitting on me in that club, the night Zeus got the scar on his eyebrow.

"You're choking him," I say with urgency as the guy gasps for air. "Just let him go, and we can go home together. Just me and you."

I can see the war he's having in his mind. A few seconds later, his hand comes from around the guy's throat, and he drops to the floor, on his hands and knees, sucking in gulps of air.

Zeus stares down at him. His voice is low and terrifying when he says, "You ever come near Cam again, even breathe in her direction or imply some shit that you know ain't true, and I'll come after you. And there won't be a fucking soul on earth who'll be able to stop me. Do you hear me?"

The pap gasps out, "I hear ya."

Zeus yanks open the passenger door. "Get in," he barks at me.

I practically jump to attention and get in the car.

Zeus is in the driver's side moments later, and then we're peeling out of there.

The anger rolling off him is palpable. It's stifling in

the confined space of his car. I feel like I'm the one choking now.

I know I should say something, but I don't know what to say.

We drive back to his apartment in that thick cloud of silence.

Zeus is still living at the apartment until his lease is up in just over a month, and then he'll move into the house. In the meantime, he's going to start work on the house, getting it ready—a new kitchen fitted, decorating the place up, buying furniture, basically making it a home.

Zeus said he wants my input on the decor, as it's my home, too, and I'll be living there soon enough, so I should like how it looks. I didn't argue with the "soon enough" comment because I know Zeus and how he gets when he sets something in his mind. Truthfully, the more I think about living with him, about us finally being a family, the more I feel comfortable with the idea—maybe even a little excited.

Though, right now, excitement is the last thing I'm feeling. Worry, trepidation . . . yep, definitely feeling those.

He parks the car outside his building. Turns off the engine. But makes no move to get out of the car.

He's sitting there. Hands curled around the steering wheel, eyes staring straight ahead.

I unclip my seat belt and shift in my seat to face him. "Zeus," I softly say his name.

"I wanted to hurt him." Dark eyes turn to mine. "I really wanted to fucking hurt him."

"I know," I say quietly. "And you did hurt him. You

hurt his pride. I'm pretty sure you broke his camera. And you definitely scared the shit out of him."

I smile, but he doesn't react. The smile fades from my face.

"After what happened with Scott"—he blows out a breath—"things started to look different. The hunger to fight . . . it didn't seem so important anymore. But then . . . in that moment, that asshole was Marcel along with every fucking journalist out there who's said something bad about you. He was every regret and mistake I've made with you. He was five years without you. He was missing out on Gigi's start in life."

My eyes fill with tears, and I reach for his hand.

"I wanted to hurt him, Cam . . . but I wanted to hurt myself more."

"Zeus . . ."

"You're better off without me," he says. "I should never have come back."

A tear spills down my cheek. "Is this you giving up on us again?"

"No." Remorseful eyes move to mine. "But you should give up on me. I'm no good for you, Dove. I'm no good for anyone."

I climb over the console, straddling his lap, and take his face in my hands. "Bullshit. You listen to me, Zeus Kincaid. I have loved you for nine years. Five of them, I spent without you, and not once did my feelings for you diminish or stop. You are good for me. We're only good together. This is just another bump in the road for us. We've gotten over bigger. And we'll get over this one."

His eyes that are fixed on mine slowly blink once. "I love you," he rasps out. "So fucking much, it hurts."

I kiss his scarred brow, then his cheek, and finally his mouth. "It hurts to love you, too, Zeus. But it also heals me. Loving you is everything."

"Fuck," he groans. His fingers plunge into my hair, and his mouth takes mine in a deep kiss. "I just wish you could see my feelings for you, Dove. See how fucking deep they run."

"So, take me inside your apartment, and show me," I whisper into his mouth.

And he does exactly that.

Zeus takes me into his apartment, and he spends the rest of the night showing me with his body just how deep his feelings for me really do go.

Chapter Thirty-Four

GIGI, ZEUS, AND I are having a lazy Saturday afternoon at his apartment.

I took Gigi shopping this morning. It'd been a while since we had our girlie time together. And then we grabbed three takeout burritos for lunch and brought them with us to eat at Zeus's place.

We're all fed up with burritos, and now, we're sitting on the sofa together, watching *Tangled* for what is quite possibly the thousandth time.

Gigi is sprawled all over Zeus like a blanket. He looks so content, sitting there with her. They both do.

It makes my heart swell. I could sit and watch them all day long like this.

Zeus catches me staring. I don't look away. It's so much easier that I don't have to hide my feelings from him or myself anymore.

The corner of his lips lifts into that stunning smile. I smile, too.

He parts his lips, wetting them with his tongue.

My sex clenches.

Down, girl. We're rated PG at the moment.

His eyes flicker down to Gigi, whose eyes are glued to the TV screen. Then, he looks back to me.

I love you, he mouths.

My smile widens so big, I'm sure my face is about to crack.

I'm just about to mouth the same words back when there's a knock at his door.

Both our eyes turn in that direction.

"You expecting anyone?" I ask him.

He shakes his head. He goes to move, but I tell him to stay put.

"I'll get it," I say, so he doesn't have to disturb Gigi.

I push up to my feet and pad barefoot to his door.

I check the peephole, and when I see who it is, a bad feeling drops into my stomach.

I unlock the door and pull it open. "Rich, Emilio," I greet them.

Emilio is also an officer at the station, and they're both in uniform, which means they're on the job. My bad feeling sinks lower.

"Everything okay?"

"Is Zeus here?" Rich asks me.

"Um . . . yeah. He's just in the living room with Gigi." I protectively hold the door close to me. "Why?"

"We just need a word with him, Cam," Emilio says.

I hear footsteps behind me. Then, Zeus's hands are pressing gently down on my shoulders but in a possessive manner.

I don't miss Rich's eyes going to them.

"What can I do for you, boys?" Zeus says.

At the term *boys*, Rich straightens up to his full height, which is still nowhere near as big as Zeus.

Testosterone. The cause of most of the world's problems.

"There's been a complaint of assault and malicious destruction of property made against you, and we need you to come to the station with us," Rich tells him.

"What?" I gasp.

The paparazzi guy.

"And you're here to take me in?" Zeus says calmly.

"No," I say, panicked. I turn my eyes to him.

He must see the fear in them because he says, "It's okay, Cam."

"No, it's not!" My voice rises in panic, and I internally chastise myself. I don't want Gigi to come here and see what's going on.

I step forward a little, toward Rich and Emilio, but Zeus doesn't relinquish his hold on me.

"Isn't there something you can do?" I plead to Rich.

Rich gives me a sad look. He shakes his head. "It's out of my hands." He reaches for the handcuffs from his belt.

Tears spring to my eyes.

Zeus moves around me, shielding me. And I instantly see Rich and Emilio stiffen.

Zeus holds his hands up in surrender. "Gigi's here," he says directly to Rich, a surprising quietness to his voice. "I'll come quietly. I'm not gonna make a scene. I just don't want my daughter to see me in those." He nods at the cuffs in Rich's hand.

Rich glances at Emilio, who nods.

Rich clips the cuffs back on his belt. "Okay," he says. "But we have to go now."

Zeus turns to me and takes my face in his hands. "I love you, and I'll be home soon," he tells me. "Tell Gigi . . . just tell her I'll be back real soon."

The ache in his eyes brings the tears back to my eyes. He firmly kisses me on the lips before I can start bawling.

I hold on to him tight, not wanting to let him go. Breathing him in, like I'm never going to see him again.

I'm going to see him again.

"I love you," I whisper against his lips.

He pulls away from me, leaving me cold, and walks out the door, past Rich and Emilio, who immediately follow him, but I catch sight of the hurt in Rich's eyes before he turns to leave.

Rich and I were never together properly, but he did have feelings for me, and I did for him to a certain degree even if he did let Zeus run him off so easily. But it's hard to care about his feelings right now when he's putting Zeus in the back of his patrol car and shutting the door.

My heart is beating like a drum against my chest.

He's coming back, Cam. It's going to be okay.

"Mommy, why is Daddy going in a *powice* car with *Wich*?"

The sound of Gigi's voice beside me has me shutting my fears away and clearing my expression. I reach down and pick her up. She wraps her legs around my waist, her arms around my neck.

"Daddy's just helping Rich with something."

"Daddy a *powiceman* now?" Her eyes light up.

"No." I kiss her hair. "He's just helping Rich with some questions; that's all. Nothing to worry about."

I watch the car pull away, catching sight of Zeus in the backseat of the police car. His eyes on me and Gigi.

And my heart starts to hurt.

Closing the front door, I turn my face to Gigi, painting on a bright smile. "How about we bake some cookies for Daddy to have when he gets home?"

"*Chocowate* chip?" She smiles hopefully.

"How does double chocolate chip sound?"

"Yay!" She excitedly claps her hands.

"I just need to call Granny Elle real quick. Why don't you go watch *Tangled* for a few more minutes, and then we can go to the store to buy the ingredients, as I'm sure Daddy doesn't have any?" I smile at her.

"Okay, Mommy," she says cheerfully. Blissfully unaware that her father is currently on his way to the police station for assaulting a paparazzo. And the arresting officer is a guy I used to sleep with.

God, what a clusterfuck of a mess.

The only consistent and sure thing in my life is this little girl in my arms. And the fact that, no matter what, I love Zeus, and I always will.

I put Gigi to her feet, and she runs off to the living room. I wait until I hear the sounds of *Tangled* resume before I slide my cell from my jeans pocket and speed-dial Aunt Elle's cell.

She answers on the second ring. "I literally just heard about the complaint filed against Zeus," she tells me, before I get a chance to say anything. "I'll deal with it, Cam. Don't worry about anything."

"Thank you," I breathe, blinking back tears from my eyes.

"Mommy! Can we go to the store yet? I wanna make *cwookies*!" Gigi calls from the living room.

"One more minute," I call to Gigi. "Sorry," I say to Aunt Elle. "I told Gigi we'd make Zeus some cookies for when he got home. I have to take her to the store—" A sob catches in my throat. I press my hand to my mouth.

"It is going to be okay, Cam. Say it."

I take a deep breath, blinking back tears. "It's going to be okay."

"Good girl. Now, you and Gigi get to baking those cookies, and I'll have Zeus back home before they've cooled."

"Thank you," I say again.

"You never need to thank me. There isn't a thing in this world that I wouldn't do for you or our Gigi girl."

Emotion clogs my throat. "I love you, Mom," I say, surprising myself.

That's the first time I've ever called her it. I don't know why I just did now. Or why I haven't always called her it.

There's a pause.

I don't know what she's thinking, and that scares me. A lump fixes in my throat, and my damp hand clamps tight around my phone.

"Should I not have said that?" I whisper.

She makes a choked sound. And, when she speaks, her voice is thick, "You're my daughter, Cam. You always have been. You always will be. Hearing you call me Mom . . ." Another pained sound comes from her.

I've never seen her cry before. She's the strongest woman I've ever known. But I'm pretty sure she is or is close to tears right now.

A tear rolls down my cheek. I brush it away. "I didn't mean to upset you."

She lets out what seems to be a happy sound. "You haven't upset me. Far from it. You've . . . I'm just happy right now. I'd rank this as the second happiest day of my life."

"What was your first?"

"The day you came to live with me and the day Gigi was born."

"That's two things," I say.

"Joint first," she tells me. "I'm not going to choose between my girls."

I laugh softly, as another tear slips down my cheek. I brush it away.

"Now, let's stop before you have me bawling, and I wreck my reputation as the station's hard-ass. Let me get Zeus out of this trouble he's gotten himself into."

"Okay," I whisper.

We hang up, and I push my cell back into my jeans pocket. I dry my face with my hands, blow out a strengthening breath, step back into Mommy mode, and walk through into the living room to find my girl sprawled out on the sofa, singing along to *Tangled*.

"Okay, Gigi girl." I clap my hands together, getting her attention. "Let's go to the store, and then we can get our bake on."

Chapter Thirty-Five

TRUE TO HER WORD, Aunt Elle got Zeus home. It took a bit longer than the time it took Gigi and I to go to the store and back and bake the cookies, but she got him home nonetheless.

Aunt Elle had Zeus released on a DAT—Desk Appearance Ticket. Meaning he wouldn't have to stay in jail until his arraignment. He's supposed to go in front of a judge in a few days, so he can be formally charged with assault and malicious destruction of property.

I know. I want to cry every time I think about it.

But Zeus is confident that it'll never get that far. And Aunt Elle agrees with him.

The paparazzi guy will want money. That's all he'll want, according to Zeus. That's why he pressed charges in the first place.

Zeus's lawyers are currently prepping to make a deal with this guy. If he accepts, which Zeus says he will, the charges will be dropped, and Zeus will pay him damages.

Sickens me to think that this guy can harass us

while we're out together, take our pictures, and say some awful, derogatory, and untruthful things about me, and Zeus is the one who has to pay. Literally.

But it's the way of the world, Zeus said.

I'm just starting to think the world sucks an awful lot more than I realized. Well, at least the world Zeus is a part of.

I'm at work, at my desk, when my cell rings. The name of the man of the moment lights up my screen, like he knew I was just thinking about him.

"Hey," I answer. "I was just thinking about you," I echo my thoughts.

"Were you thinking about the amazing things I could do to you with my tongue?"

"I wasn't, but I am now." I squirm in my seat.

"So, how about you come to my apartment on your lunch break, and I can do those things to you in celebration of the asshole dropping the charges?"

"Really?"

"Really," he says. "I just got the call from my lawyer. I have to pay the asshole fifty thousand dollars, but—"

"Fifty thousand dollars!" I shriek, quickly glancing around to make sure nobody heard me.

"It's fine."

"No, it's not. You shouldn't have to pay fifty thousand dollars to that asshole."

"Dove, I'd pay it twice if it meant I got to shut him up again. It's not a big deal. It's only money. Just let it go. I have. And come here and celebrate the charges going away with me in bed."

I draw in a deep breath and let it out. "Okay. But I'm

the one who's going to be doing the amazing things with my tongue to you. You deserve it."

He growls, and it makes me shiver.

"I'm not gonna argue with that. How long till your lunch break?"

I glance up at the clock on the wall. "Just under an hour."

"Can you leave sooner?"

"I wish."

"Then, I'll see you and that sexy mouth of yours in less than an hour."

I hang up the phone with a smile on my face, feeling a lot less stressed than I did five minutes ago and a heck of a lot more excited about my lunch break than usual.

I pull my car up in front of Zeus's building, parking behind a big-ass black SUV.

I check my teeth in the rearview mirror, smooth my hair down, and sort the girls' position in my bra, making sure I've got ample cleavage showing. Grab my perfume from my bag and spritz myself with it.

Ready, I hang my bag on my shoulder and exit my car. I lock it and walk toward Zeus's apartment.

I get the key he gave me to his place from my bag and let myself in. I hear the sound of male voices the moment I push the door open.

Huh? He has guests? What happened to my smexy lunchtime?

I close the door behind me and walk down the hall and into the living room.

The first thing I see is the less than welcome sight of

Marcel Duran sitting in the middle of the sofa and two burly-looking guys standing on either side of it.

Oh, fucking fuck. What the hell is he doing here?

My eyes quickly seek out Zeus, who's seated on the arm of the chair across from Marcel, hands clenched into fists on his thighs, staring at Marcel like he's seconds away from killing him.

Jesus Christ. His lawyer only just got the charges for assault dropped this morning. The last thing I need is him killing Marcel and his cronies.

"Zeus," I say quietly.

Zeus's eyes flick to mine, the surprise in them telling me that he's only just registered my being here. But, behind the surprise, I see the undiluted rage.

If I thought he was angry with that paparazzi guy the other day, then I was wrong. He was clearly just playing then in comparison to the way he looks right now.

"Cameron!" Marcel exclaims my name like it's a production, spreading his arms wide. "It's been so long since I last saw you."

"Not long enough," I say before I can stop myself.

Marcel chortles like I was joking. I wasn't.

Zeus pushes to his feet. "Marcel was just leaving."

"What? Come on now, Zeus. I only just got here," he says cheerfully. "It's been a while since we saw each other. We have a lot to catch up on. And there's some business we need to discuss before I go. Now, be a love, Cameron, and go make me a coffee. I take it black, two sugars. Matt, Earl, you want anything?" he asks his paid lackeys, who have a vague resemblance to Ren and Stimpy.

"She's not your fucking waitress," Zeus snaps.

Annoyance flickers through Marcel's eyes. But it's gone as quickly as it arrived.

"My apologies, Cameron. I didn't mean to offend," Marcel says without a lick of sincerity in his words.

Zeus moves in front of me, blocking me from view. His arms curl around my upper arms. "Go back to work. I'll call you as soon as I'm done."

"No," I whisper. "I'm not leaving you alone here." I try to convey my meaning with my eyes. As in, *I daren't leave you here with him in case you lose your shit and hit him and then end up at the police station again.* Somehow, I can't see a payoff of fifty grand satisfying Marcel.

"Cam . . ." Zeus says my name low and with meaning.

"Let her stay, Zeus," Marcel says sounding suddenly bored.

Zeus turns to face him, keeping me partially concealed behind him. "How about you say what you came here to say, and then you leave?"

Marcel sighs. Pushes himself forward in his seat. His hands resting on his knees. "Well, I wouldn't have had to come here if you'd answered my calls."

"There was a reason I wasn't answering your calls. The same fucking reason you shouldn't be here right now. Because I'm still figuring out how not to wrap my hands around your throat and choke the life out of you."

Marcel's beady eyes darken. "You threatening me, Zeus? Because that'd be a real stupid move to make."

Zeus's step toward Marcel is menacing. My hand hangs on to the back of his T-shirt, like I'd somehow be able to stop him if he decided to go for him.

The Ren and Stimpy lookalikes make a point of stepping forward, too.

Zeus looks at them both and smirks before taking his eyes back to Marcel. "I'm not threatening you, Duran. I'm simply stating a fact." Zeus's voice is eerily calm, sending shivers down my spine. "And, really, these guys? You brought these for protection? I could take them both down without even breaking a sweat, and you know it."

"I also know you wouldn't do jack shit because you care too much about your little family to risk screwing things up, and I'm not talking about the family that she tricked you into having. I'm talking about that kid brother and sister of yours who are still in college, relying on you to keep them there. And don't forget your dad and his love of the bottle. How many rehab visits is that now, Zeus?"

"Tricked him?" I exclaim, letting my bag slide from my shoulder and to the floor. "The only one who tricked Zeus into anything was you, you crazy bastard! When you made him believe he would be better off without me!"

Okay, so maybe it's me that's going to lose my shit by staying here.

Marcel laughs and gets to his feet. It sounds like a laugh Santa would make. But that man is far from Santa. More like Satan. "Honey, I didn't need to make him believe anything. He couldn't wait to get away from you and into all the pussy waiting for him."

I actually see red. I didn't know that was a real thing. Apparently, it is. I want blood. Specifically, Marcel Duran's.

I make a lunge for him, but Zeus catches me around the waist, preventing me from going anywhere. And I'm like a cat fighting to get free.

"Cam. Stop," Zeus rasps low into my ear, yanking me back to the now.

Marcel laughs the most patronizing sound I've ever heard. "You need to keep your woman under control, Zeus. This was always the problem with her. Overly emotional. Getting in your head all the time. Distracting you and dragging you down."

"The only one who dragged me down was you." Zeus glares at him.

"Drag you down? I made you, Kincaid. You'd do well to remember that. You'd be fighting in pool halls with an audience size that I could count on my hands, spending your days still working in that shithole factory to make ends meet, if it wasn't for me."

It's Zeus's turn to laugh. "You keep telling yourself that, Duran. Did you forget I was already an Olympic champion and that I had a Golden Gloves win under my belt when you came knocking at my door?"

"You had nothing. A gold medal and an amateur boxing title that means jack shit in the actual world of boxing. I put you where you are, Zeus, and don't you forget it."

"You did nothing! It was me in that ring, winning every fight! Me training every fucking day. Sweat, blood, and fucking pain!" He slams a hand to his chest. "I was the one who sacrificed the person who mattered most to me because you'd made me believe it was the only way! Because of you, I lost the first four years of my daughter's life!"

Marcel actually has the audacity to sigh and roll his eyes. "You have your daughter now, so what's the big deal? I did you a favor, not telling you that she was knocked up. If you'd known, you would've come running back to her, and you wouldn't be where you are right now."

"Where I am right now?" Zeus laughs a disbelieving sound. "Right now, I'm here, fighting to get my family back with me, all because of the damage you did."

"And there it is." Marcel spreads his arms wide. "Blame me all you want. But the problem is her." He points a fat finger at me. "It has always been her. Do you think I would've had to keep her pregnancy from you if she hadn't been up in your ear all the time, fucking with your head, making you think that the only important thing in your life was her?"

"She was the only important thing in my life!" Zeus roars.

"If that's true, then you wouldn't have walked away from her so easily."

I feel sick at those words. Because those are the exact words that rattle around in the back of my brain all the damn time.

"Yeah, easy—that's what it was, Marcel," Zeus scoffs. "Not one fucking thing about walking away from Cam was easy for me, and you knew it."

"After she was gone, you became the fighter you were always meant to be. I did you a favor."

"Am I supposed to thank you for ruining my life?"

"Don't be so fucking melodramatic. You've been spending too much time around her again."

"I fucking hate you," I hiss at him.

He laughs that chortling, annoying-as-hell laugh. "You're not the first, sweetheart, and you sure as hell won't be the last. I'm not in this business to make friends."

"No. But you were supposed to look out for me," Zeus says with an edge to his voice.

"I did."

"No!" Zeus roars. "You looked out for yourself! I gave Cam up to give Ares, Lo, and Missy a shot at a decent future because you made me believe that it was the only way it would happen!

"*No outside distractions, Kincaid. Don't take her calls, Kincaid. You think she's waiting around for you at that ballet school in New York? Hell no. She's spending her time with those artsy-fartsy male dancers. You don't need that shit in your head. A clear mind equals a better fighter. Do you think Ali or Frazier sat around, fretting over their girlfriends? No. They cut that shit loose, and they got in the ring and did what they had to do.*" Zeus mimics Marcel's voice.

"You were in my head all the fucking time. And I listened to you because I trusted you. I thought, putting all the bullshit and bravado aside, that you had my best interests at heart. But that was a lie. The only thing you've ever cared about is the numbers on the check that you've banked after every fight I did for you.

"I should've listened to Cam when she told me in the beginning that she didn't have a great feeling about you. But I didn't listen to her. I won't make that mistake again. Now, get the fuck out of my apartment before I do something neither of us will be able to come back from."

Marcel's face is blank. Expressionless.

He puts a hand inside his jacket and pulls out a brown envelope.

He drops it on the coffee table in front of him. "Your training schedule and details for the Dimitrov fight. It's set for six weeks from now. So, you'd better start training. Because, if you lose this fight, Zeus, I will take every cent you have, and I won't stop until you and your entire family, including her and that kid of yours, are sleeping in a dumpster."

I expect Zeus to argue. Say he's not doing the fight. Tell him to fuck off in the very least. But he doesn't. He just stares Marcel in the eyes and nods his head once in agreement.

My insides flare up like gasoline poured on a bonfire. I have to bite my tongue hard to stop from saying anything.

But I will not discuss this with Zeus in front of Marcel. I won't give the asshole the satisfaction.

I watch with gritted teeth as Marcel and his posse head for the door.

"Just one thing before you go." Zeus turns his head to look at Marcel. "Was it you who gave the press the bullshit story on Cam?"

Marcel smiles, and I want to wipe the smug look off his ugly face.

"What do I always say to you, Zeus? There are two rules in life. The first is, never give out all the information." He pats a hand to the door and walks out of it.

I stare after him, mouth open. "That's it?" I say angrily when I hear the telltale slam of the front door, whirling around to Zeus. "What the hell is that supposed to mean?"

"It means he covered his ass by feeding yours to the press. No one would believe he did what he did if we came out and told everyone after your story broke. It would have looked like a weak attempt at passing off the blame to clear your name."

"That man is the actual devil."

Zeus doesn't respond to that. He just sighs and goes over to the chair where he sits down, putting his head into his hands.

I sit down on the coffee table and pick up the envelope. "Please tell me you're not actually going to go ahead with this fight."

He lowers his hands, eyes coming to meet mine. "We've been over this before, Cam. I don't have a choice."

"There's always a choice."

"Not this time." He shakes his head.

I push up to my feet. "I can't believe you're still going to work with that guy after what he did to us."

Zeus stands. "You think I like it any more than you do? No. But I'm contractually bound. If I walk away from that fight, I will lose everything I've worked for."

"So, this is about money?"

"Yes. Of course it is. Do you think I'm doing this for fun? If I had my way, I would bury Marcel back in the hole that he first crawled out of, but right now, until I do this fight, it's not an option."

"Is money the only thing that matters to you?" I hate myself for saying it the second I do because I know that's not true.

His expression darkens. "You and Gigi and Ares,

Lo, and Missy are the only things that matter to me. And to give you the lives you deserve means I have to earn money. And I do that in the only way I know how. I fight, Cam. It's what I do. It's what I'm good at. It's who I am!" He slams a hand to his chest.

"That's not just who you are!" I counter. "You're a father and a brother and a son to a man who doesn't deserve you. And you're . . . mine, Zeus. My best friend. My partner. The love of my life. And I don't care about the money. Gigi doesn't care about the money. We can figure something out with Lo and Missy finishing college. Ares could help. I'm sure the NFL is paying him well."

"He already pays half of their tuition fees," Zeus admits to me.

"So, what's the problem then? I'm sure he could cover the whole of it until they graduate. And your dad . . . well, let him stand on his own two feet for once in his life."

Zeus turns from me, his hands going to the back of his neck, fingers linking together. I hear him expel a harsh breath.

I walk up behind him and press my hand to his back. "What aren't you telling me?"

His arms come down from his neck, and he turns to face me. The look in his eyes has my pulse jumping with worry of what he might be about to say.

"I know you don't care about the money," he says in a quiet voice. "But I need Gigi's future to be secure, Dove. I want her to have every opportunity that money can afford. Every opportunity that I never had. And, no matter what my dad has done or how much he's let us down . . . he's my dad. I can't just leave him to fend for himself."

"And?"

He briefly closes his eyes before opening them. "And . . . there's another reason I need the money."

"Which is?"

He stares at me for a long moment, guilt and shame swimming in his beautiful eyes. "Kaden Scott," he says low and pained. "I need the money for Kaden Scott."

Chapter Thirty-Six

"I DON'T UNDERSTAND. WHY WOULD you need money for Kaden?"

"To pay for his ongoing treatment and living assistance. He's in a fucking wheelchair, Cam. He might not walk again."

"I understand that, but does his insurance not cover it?"

"Not the level of treatment and physio that he deserves. And he doesn't have any family, Cam. He's all alone."

"Seriously?"

"He was raised in foster care. His so-called friends along with his manager were nowhere to be seen after his hospitalization. They all just fucking left him. Walked away without a backward glance."

"Assholes," I say, thinking how lucky I was to have Aunt Elle, or I could have ended up in foster care when my mom died.

"A lot of people are in this business. They only care about money and stature. A fighter is a paycheck to promoters, and if he's not making money, then he's worthless to them. They tossed Scott out like he was trash. He was in a bad way for a long time. I spent pretty much all of the last twelve months visiting him at the hospital. Trying to help in any way I could. I only came back to New York to start my training for the Dimitrov fight. But then I found you, and . . . everything changed."

"Where's he being treated?"

"Arizona. There's a great rehabilitation facility there. I had him moved there from the hospital in Atlantic City once he was well enough to be transported. Scott hasn't once asked me for a dime. He didn't ask for my help. It was only when I was there, visiting, that I overheard a conversation he was having with his doctor, regarding his options for treatment. He hates that I'm paying for his treatment and insists that he'll pay me every dime back—stubborn bastard that he is. But I put him there, Cam. Paying for his treatment and care and being his friend—it's the very fucking least I can do."

"I don't think it was your fault, Zeus. You all get in that ring, knowing the dangers, but I do understand why you feel responsible and want to help him."

"That's why I need the money from the Dimitrov fight. It's big fucking money, Cam. It'll enable me to help Scott for as long as he needs. But it'll also secure Gigi's future."

I stare at the wall behind him, hating that he feels he has to do this but understanding why. "Why didn't you tell me before now?"

He drags his hand down his face. "Because I was ashamed. I *am* ashamed. Scott's in this position because of me. I knew something wasn't right. I should've stopped the fight."

"No. That's what referees are for. It's not on you to stop the fight."

"It was my fist that hit him hard enough to make his head snap back, rupturing an artery, causing a blood clot on his brain. I'm the reason he stopped breathing and lost oxygen to the brain for more minutes than acceptable. Multiple surgeries, a stroke, a fucking wheelchair. Cam . . . I did that to him. He's my responsibility."

I close my eyes at the bluntness of what he's saying.

"I understand . . ." I say, opening my eyes. "But I think you're being too hard on yourself."

"I'm not being hard enough. I have everything here. I have you back. I have Gigi, my kid brothers and sister, and even my dad. Scott has nothing and no one, except for me and the doctors treating him and the nurses caring for him. His whole life changed. His future, everything he could've been, was taken from him with one single punch."

"And, now, to help him, you're going to fight someone else, risk the same thing happening again." I wrap my arms around myself at the thought, trying to ward off the chill it brings.

"Dimitrov isn't a guy you need to worry about. What happened to Scott won't happen to him. The guy's head is made out of stone."

"It's not him I'm worried about getting hurt!" I exclaim. "It's you!"

Zeus frowns, taking my words like an insult. Like I think he's weak. I don't think he's weak. But I think

Dimitrov is unpredictable. I've read and heard the stories about him.

"He won't get near me," Zeus grinds the words out.

"He's an animal, who has no concept of the rules. He should be in a cage. Not a boxing ring."

Zeus takes my face in his hands. "He won't get near me," he enunciates. "I've never lost a fight. In all these years, no one has gotten close to hurting me."

I point to the scar on his brow. "The guy who did that got close, real close, to hurting you."

"A bar fight with a glass bottle is a helluva lot different than two gloved guys in a boxing ring."

I heave out a sigh, knowing that his mind is set, and nothing I say or do will make him see things differently.

"Dove"—he cups my chin with his hand—"promise me that you won't worry about this."

I move my eyes to his. "I can't promise that."

"Cam . . ."

I pull from his hold. "Don't ask me not to worry about you, okay? I love you. It comes with the territory. I get why you need to do this, why you feel that you need to do the fight with that crazy bastard Dimitrov, but it doesn't mean that I have to like it. I just . . . I need some time to get my head around it, so . . ." I take a small step back. "I'm going to go back to work. My lunch break is almost over anyway."

I lean forward and give him a quick, perfunctory kiss on the cheek. Then, I cross the room and pick my bag up from the floor, hanging it on my shoulder.

"Dove . . ."

I stop by the door and glance back at him.

"Are we going to be okay?" he asks in a quiet voice.

I give him a small smile. "We're gonna be fine," I tell him.

Because it's true. It's not *us* that I'm worried about. It's him stepping into that ring with Dimitrov that has me running scared.

Chapter Thirty-Seven

Four Weeks Later

"MOMMY." THE SOUND OF Gigi's whispering voice rouses me from a deep sleep.

"You okay, Gigi girl?" I mumble.

"Uh-huh. But why's Daddy *sweeping* in your bed?"

My eyes flash open to see Zeus lying facedown, fast asleep beside me, his strong arm slung over my stomach, pinning me there. The duvet is fortunately covering what I know is his bare ass.

Oh, fuck.

Fucking fuck.

He stayed last night after Gigi went to bed. We haven't had much alone time since he started training for his fight.

Do I feel better about his upcoming fight? No. But I'm dealing. Kind of.

When Zeus trains, it's intense. He's hardly here at the moment, and when he is, he rightly spends time with Gigi. Meaning sex has been sparse—okay, nonexistent this last month. But he was all frisky last night, and who was I to say no? Especially not when he threw me down on the bed and went down on me, giving me the orgasm to top all orgasms. Then, we ended up fucking like animals for the next hour, and we must've passed out from exhaustion because he's still here. And Gigi's seen us together in bed, and—*Crap . . . am I naked, too?*

My hand glides up from its place on the bed, and I'm relieved to feel my nightshirt, which I now remember putting on before Zeus talked me into cuddling for a few minutes before he was supposed to leave to go home to the house, which he is now living in, as his lease was up on his apartment.

"He's, um . . . well, Daddy was tired, and I said he could sleep here, so . . ."

"Why's Daddy gots no clothes on?"

Fucking, fucking fuck.

"Um . . . because . . . because . . ."

"Because I get hot in bed, Gigi girl." He reaches over and grabs her, pulling her onto the bed between us, making her giggle and squeal. "And I'm not naked. I'm wearing shorts. See?" He lifts the cover, showing her his running shorts, which he was wearing last night.

But I'm now wondering when he put those on because I distinctly remember him being naked when we were lying here, cuddling, before we fell asleep.

And, now, I'm wondering if he fell asleep here on purpose, so Gigi would find him here and know that we were together. He's not asked me directly to tell Gigi that we're together, but he has recently been making definite noises in that direction.

I stare at him, brow lifted, but he doesn't look at me, so I poke him in the arm with my finger.

He glances at me, and I give him a questioning look.

"What?" he says.

"When did you put those on?" I nod in the general vicinity of his shorts.

"Don't know. Must've done it in my sleep."

"Uh-huh." I nod. "Sure you did."

He gives me a look of innocence, which I one hundred percent do not believe.

"So, will Daddy *sweep* here all the time now?"

"No," I'm quick to answer.

Zeus gives me a less than impressed look. "But if I were to"—he moves his eyes back to Gigi—"how would you feel about that?"

"Good 'cause then you'd be here all the times."

My heart clenches hard, like she just put her little hand around it and squeezed it tight.

"So, if I said to you that me and Daddy were together now, would that be okay with you?" I ask her.

"Together?" Her eyes and cute button nose screw up with confusion.

"Like Rapunzel and Flynn Ryder," I explain. "A couple."

"Ohs, like boyfriends and girlfriends?" She beams.

"Yeah, like boyfriend and girlfriend."

"I *finks* that'd be awesome." She pauses, looking between me and Zeus, her nose screwing up again. "But you's not gonna be kissing all the time, are you?"

Zeus barks out a laugh, and I go beet red.

"No! Of course not. Where on earth did you get that from?" I ask her.

"T.V." She shrugs.

"What do you mean, TV?" I ask her.

"Movies, Mommy." She gives me a look that says this should be perfectly obvious. "The mans and womens are always kissing in the movies."

She starts to make kissing sounds, and Zeus laughs again, harder this time.

"And no more movies for you." I reach over and tickle her side, making her squirm and giggle.

Looks like I'm going to have to monitor even more closely exactly what it is she's watching on the television.

"Daddy?"

"Yes, Gigi."

"Does this mean that you and Mommy are gonna gets *mwarried*?"

"No!" I say at the exact same time that Zeus says, "Yeah. One day."

My eyes snap to Zeus, who's staring back at me, a furrow puckering his brow.

I move my eyes from him to Gigi. "We won't be getting married anytime soon," I say to Gigi.

"Okay." She sighs. Another pause and then, "But, when you do's gets *mwarried*, I be a bridesmaids, right?"

A smile creeps onto my face. I glance over at Zeus to see he's grinning, too.

I press a kiss to her soft hair and say, "If Mommy and Daddy ever get married, you'll be the only bridesmaid, Gigi girl."

"*Pwomise*?"

"I promise."

She goes quiet again. I've just closed my eyes, and I'm dozing, loving just being here with my little family, when her little voice breaks the quiet.

"Mommy?"

"Yes, Gigi girl?"

"Can we all gets up and watch TV together now?"

"What do you want to watch?" Zeus asks her on a yawn.

"*Tangled*, of *cwourse*."

Sigh.

Chapter Thirty-Eight

"LADIES AND GENTLEMEN, I want you on your feet. It's been too long since we last saw him in the ring . . . so be upstanding to welcome your very own homegrown champion . . . Zeus . . . 'The God' . . . Kincaid!"

The crowd goes wild. Zeus's boxing anthem, "Lose Yourself," starts to thrum through the stadium.

My eyes pull up to one of the big screens. It shows Zeus coming through the stadium, making his way to the ring. His robe on, hood up, face composed, focused.

My heart starts to pound with worry. It's hard not to feel the adrenaline buzzing through the stadium, feel the rush of people's excitement. But I'm scared. Because the guy about to climb into that ring with a complete psycho is the man I love. The father of my child.

Thankfully, Gigi won't see this. She's at home with Aunt Elle. She should be in bed by now. She knows that Zeus has a boxing match tonight, but thankfully, she doesn't really understand what that means.

I'm here with Ares, Lo, and Missy, and we're seated in the front row.

Close enough that I'll be able to hear every punch thrown.

I wince at the thought.

The tickets would have been expensive if we'd paid for them. But, when your boyfriend is the headline fighter, you get them for free.

Tonight is the big-money fight because, if Zeus wins, it means he will hold all five heavyweight division titles. They call it unifying the division.

Hence, the hefty price tag on the tickets.

When we were younger, this was something Zeus always used to say he wanted to achieve.

I recently asked him if this was one of the reasons he wanted to do the fight as well as the money. But he said no.

I don't know if he feels that he should say that because of the guilt he harbors over Kaden.

Tons of celebrities are here to watch the fight. I can't even be excited that Jake Wethers and Tom Carter from The Mighty Storm are sitting three seats away from me because I'm so nervous.

Maybe, when Zeus wins, I'll have my freak-out over them.

But all I can think about right now is Zeus, praying he comes out of this okay.

I watched all of Zeus's fights in the years we were together. I always felt nervous back then, but I can honestly say nothing compares to how I'm feeling right now.

I feel sick.

I press my hand to my stomach.

I'm afraid that he's going to get hurt. Seriously hurt.

I knew of Dimitrov from the news stories. But I made it my business to watch some of his fights. I didn't tell Zeus because he didn't want me to worry.

I'm worried.

The guy is an animal.

Think Mike Tyson on crack.

That's Roman Dimitrov.

I don't think he'd give a shit if he killed someone.

And Zeus is getting in the ring with that lunatic.

Zeus is big, and he's strong. He's in peak physical shape. He always is. And the last six weeks of intense training has brought him up to where he needs to be.

But Dimitrov is in great shape, too.

Although Zeus has the edge in weight and height, there's not much difference between them.

I turn to look at Zeus when I know he's near ringside.

His eyes find me right away. His expression might be hardened, but his eyes . . . right now, they're all for me.

He reaches the ring and jogs up the steps.

Before he enters the ropes, he looks back at me. My heart simultaneously soars and plummets because this is it. The moment I've been dreading for the last six weeks.

I love you, I mouth to him.

His lips lift into that smile of his, and my insides putter to a stop. Then, he climbs in the ring, and my insides sag to the ground.

"It's gonna be okay," Missy says, sliding her hand into mine. My eyes move to hers. "This is Zeus. He's unbeatable."

There's always a first time for everything, my fear says.

But I don't say those words.

Instead, I force a smile and say, "Yeah, you're right."

"I'm always right." She grins. "My big brother is a hard-ass. And I, for one, cannot wait to see him put Dimitrov on his own ass."

"Hell yeah!" Ares says, reaching around me and high-fiving her.

"Five rounds most, and Zeus will put him down," Lo says.

The most recognizable voice in the boxing world starts speaking from within the ring, drawing my eyes there, "And here is the moment we've all been waiting for! Our fighters are in the ring, and they are ready to go all twelve rounds! In the blue corner, coming all the way from Bulgaria . . . standing at six feet four inches and weighing in at two hundred forty-five pounds, the current WBA and IBO heavyweight champion . . . Roman . . . 'The Jawbreaker' . . . Dimitrov."

The cheers are outweighed by the boos. Ares, Lo, and Missy are shouting negativity in Dimitrov's direction.

I'm silent. Eyes pinned on Zeus.

He looks calm. Ready to fight. But calm.

"In the red corner, standing at six feet six inches and weighing in at two hundred fifty pounds, he is the IBF, WBC, and WBO world heavyweight champion . . . your homegrown fighter . . . Zeus . . . 'The God' . . . Kincaid!"

The crowd roars with applause and cheers, and I actually find my voice and cheer for my man as he lifts his arms to the crowd, moving around the ring. I cheer louder.

When the crowd hushes, the announcer says, "To the twenty thousand in attendance and the millions watching at home, ladies and gentlemen, from Madison Square Garden in New York City . . . let's . . . geeet . . . rrrreeeaaady . . . toooo . . . ruuummmble!"

I watch as they step up close with the referee between them, firing out his rules. Then, they're back to their corners.

I watch as Zeus's trainer, Mike, talks to him. Zeus nods his head. His shield is put in his mouth, and then he's on his feet.

The bell rings.

It's time.

There's no hesitation. Zeus is in the center of the ring straightaway, intimidating and dominating. And the punches start flying.

Zeus is all over Dimitrov.

He moves so quickly, ducking every punch Dimitrov throws, leaving him punching air.

I can see the frustration building in Dimitrov's face.

And from what I saw of his previous fights, if things aren't going Dimitrov's way, like a bad loser, he starts fighting dirty.

Bell rings, signaling the end of round one, and they each go back to their corner.

But I can't relax. I'm on the edge of my seat. I just need Zeus to knock Dimitrov out, so this can be over, and I can take him home and hold him for the rest of the night. And the rest of for ever.

The bell signals round two.

Dimitrov comes out fighting and lands a punch on Zeus.

I suck in a sharp breath, shutting my eyes on the impact. But not for long because I need to know that Zeus is okay.

He is. The blow didn't even break his stride. If anything, it's fired him up.

Bang. Bang. Bang.

He has Dimitrov on the ropes.

The referee separates them. Then, it's back on.

It goes this way for three rounds.

And I've found my voice, shouting encouragement to Zeus along with Ares, Lo, and Missy. My throat will be hoarse by the end of the night, but I don't care.

I want Zeus to know I'm in his corner.

Round five.

There's a shift in the dynamics. It's almost like Dimitrov took a hit of coke, because he comes from that corner like a bull out of a cage. He's on Zeus, punch after punch, and Zeus is blocking only half of them.

Zeus's back hits the ropes, and the referee pulls them apart.

"Come on, baby!" I scream. "Knock the bastard on his psychotic ass!"

I hear the rumble of Ares's laughter from beside me. I glance at him, and he's grinning at me.

"What?"

"Nothing." He smirks. "Just having flashbacks to Zeus's early fights. You always did have a potty mouth."

"Just showing my support." I grin innocently.

"I'm glad he has you back," he says in a quieter voice.

My grin softens to a smile. "Me, too." I press my hand to his arm and give it a gentle squeeze.

The negative sound of the crowd whirls my eyes back

to Zeus. I see it like it happens in slow motion—Dimitrov's fist retracting back from Zeus's face. Zeus staggers back a step and then drops to his hands and knees.

"Noooo!" I cry, my heart free-falling, as I rush forward to the railings separating the crowd from the ring, wanting to vault over them and go to him.

Missy is there beside me. Her arm around me. Then, Ares and Lo are there. They're yelling, but I can't hear what they're saying. Blood is roaring in my ears.

Dimitrov is walking around the ring, arms in the air, like he's won.

The referee is down on his knees, beside Zeus, his mouth at his ear, talking to Zeus.

Get up, baby, please.

A second later, Zeus pushes back up onto his knees. The referee stands. And then Zeus jumps up to his feet.

And I breathe again.

The referee moves to the center of the ring. Zeus and Dimitrov are about to go in again, but the bell rings.

Zeus turns back to his corner, and there's blood running down his cheek.

No.

"He's hurt," I say to Ares.

"It's just a cut. He'll be fine."

"Has this happened before?" I ask.

In Zeus's fights that I watched when we were younger, no one could get close enough to hit him hard enough to cut him. He's had his nose broken. But I've never seen his skin split from a hit—except for that time in the club, and that guy used a bottle.

Ares's eyes meet mine. If he's trying to hide his

concern, he's doing a piss-poor job of it because I can see it loud and clear.

"He broke his nose in the Scott fight, but they went eleven rounds."

We're only five in, and he's bleeding already.

Fuck. Fuck. Fuck.

My eyes flash back to Zeus, who's on the stool in his corner, his eye being tended to. Vaseline is being rubbed around the wound to curb the bleeding. A member of his team squirts water into his mouth.

The bell goes.

Round six.

Zeus goes in, blazing.

Hitting Dimitrov with a body shot from his left. A punch to the head with his right. Another. And another.

He pounds into Dimitrov, forcing him back onto the ropes.

"Yes! Hit him, baby! Hit him!"

Dimitrov wraps his arms around Zeus's neck. The referee forces them apart.

But Zeus is straight back in, pounding into Dimitrov. Body. Face. Blow after blow.

Dimitrov stumbles back.

Zeus swings hard, connecting with his head.

The punch so audible, it seems to echo around the stadium.

Dimitrov goes down.

Zeus goes for him again, but the referee stops him, blocking him off.

Dimitrov tries to get up but can't.

The referee moves over him. His arm comes up, ending the fight.

"Yeeesss!" I scream.

The teams flood the ring.

I want in that ring. I want Zeus.

I look at Ares, and he must see it on my face as he grabs hold of me and lifts me over the barrier.

I hotfoot it to the ring, running up the steps.

"Zeus!" I cry.

His head swings around to me. He gives me that beautiful, cocky smile of his.

And I smile so big, my face might crack.

Then, I'm pushing past people to get to him. I reach him and jump into his arms, knowing that I will never leave them again.

Chapter Thirty-Nine

WE'RE IN THE DRESSING room. Just me and Zeus. The doctor just left after finishing examining the cut under Zeus's eye. Thankfully, it's not too bad. It didn't need stitches. He taped it up. But it still looks really swollen. He's going to have one hell of a black eye.

Zeus is sitting on the examination table. I'm standing between his legs, his hands resting on my hips.

"So, I have something to tell you," I say to him.

"Oh, yeah?"

"Yep."

"Good or bad?"

"I'd say, good."

"Hit me with it."

"No more hitting tonight, okay?" I quip.

He rumbles out a laugh. "No more hitting," he agrees.

"Okay." I take a fortifying breath, holding on to the courage I've been building up all day. "So, I think—"

I don't get to finish that sentence because the door

swings open, and in comes Marcel, surprisingly alone, but he doesn't close the door.

Then, I spot a security guy standing outside the door.

Zeus's whole body instantly tenses up, his grip on me tightening.

I couldn't move if I wanted to, and I don't. I want to stay exactly where I am, so hopefully, Marcel will get the message that he's not wanted, and he'll disappear.

Wishful thinking, I know.

But the fight is done. Zeus no longer has a contractual obligation to him.

"What do you want, Marcel?" Zeus barks.

"I just came to congratulate you on the win. You made us both a lot of money tonight."

"You're not welcome," Zeus dryly tosses back.

But the words just bounce off Marcel. The guy has the hide of a rhino.

"Zeus, come on. I know we've recently had our differences. But we're both man enough to see past that when there are bigger things at stake. Now that you hold all the championship titles, your value just went through the roof. If you stay with me, the fights I can bring in will make you richer than Mayweather."

Zeus laughs, not a hint of humor in it. "I'll pass, thanks."

Marcel looks at Zeus like he doesn't understand the words he just said.

"We're done here, Duran."

"Zeus, don't be stupid. We're talking hundreds of millions of dollars."

"This isn't me being stupid. This is me being smart."

Marcel's eyes flicker to me and then back to Zeus. "You're making a big mistake, Zeus. You won't fight again without me. I'll make sure of it."

Zeus tips his head to the side. "Who said I wanted to fight again?"

Marcel laughs a patronizing sound. "What are you gonna do? Sit around, being her bitch, all day long while she bleeds you dry? You're being an idiot, Kincaid."

I expect Zeus to get angry. But he doesn't. He just stares at Marcel.

Then, he starts laughing. And it's a real genuine laugh, like he's laughing at a joke that only he knows the punch line to.

"What the fuck are you laughing at?" Marcel bites, sounding rattled.

Zeus lifts his shoulder, laughter still rumbling inside his chest. "Guess you'll find out soon enough."

"What the fuck is that supposed to mean?" Marcel's beady eyes narrow into slits.

Zeus's face turns serious. "What do I always say to you, Marcel? There are two rules in life. The first is, never give out all the information."

I remember Marcel saying those exact words to Zeus six weeks ago at his apartment, and a smile creeps onto my face because I have a feeling that Zeus knows something he's not letting on about.

He previously said to me that he had something happening in the background when it came to Marcel. Maybe that's finally happening.

"You've fucking lost it," Marcel yaps as he heads for the door. "Too many hits to the head have made you even more of a dumb fuck than you already were."

"Uh-huh," Zeus says, grinning. "Piece of advice for you, Marcel. Don't bend over in the shower."

Huh? Don't bend over in the shower?

Marcel's brows crash together. "You're a fucking freak. Have a nice life with your bastard and your stripper," Marcel imparts before disappearing out of the room.

Zeus growls as he tries to move me aside and get off the examination table to get to Marcel, but I'm not budging.

"Zeus, he's not worth it," I say, gripping hold of his arms. "It doesn't matter what he says."

Zeus's brows are tight with anger.

"He only said it to get a rise out of you. If you went after him, you'd be giving him exactly what he wanted."

He exhales a sound of sheer frustration. "You're right. I know you're right. I just fucking hate him, thinking he can say whatever shit he wants about you and get away with it."

"But he's not getting away with it, is he?"

Zeus's eyes come to mine, and there's a smirk in them.

"What have you done?"

"It's not what I've done. It's what he's been doing."

I give him a look of confusion.

"Fight-fixing," he tells me in a low voice.

"No," I gasp.

"Yep." He nods.

"When? For how long? Which fighters? And how do you know?"

"That's a lot of questions, Dove." He chuckles. "And I know because Marcel isn't the only one who pokes around in other people's business. For years, I've been hearing things about him doing not-so-legal things. Fight-fixing, illegal betting syndicates—those kinds of things. But I just brushed it aside because he wasn't asking me to get involved, so it wasn't any of my business. But then, he messed around with my life, stole four years of my daughter's life from me, so I made it my business. I did some real digging. You see, the thing with Marcel is, he has a tendency to piss off a lot of people, so it's not hard to get them talking. I had a few bits of evidence but nothing solid, so I spoke to Elle—"

"Aunt Elle knows about this?" I say, surprised.

He carefully eyes me. "I asked her not to say anything until I knew there was something definite that could be done. I didn't want to drag you into it. Elle's a cop, she knows people, so she pointed me in the right direction of who I needed to speak with, and I handed off what I knew to them."

"And?"

"A couple of hours before the fight, I got a call from the detective who'd been looking into it. He told me that they would be bringing formal charges against Marcel—not just for fixing fights and illegal betting, but money laundering as well."

"Holy crap," I breathe.

"Yep. And, if he gets found guilty, he could be looking at anything up to twenty years in the state's finest."

"Well, hell," I say. "Remind me never to mess with you."

Zeus laughs before hooking his fingers into my belt loops and pulling me closer. Then, his expression turns serious. "You never have to worry about me hurting you again, Dove. I swear, I will never make that mistake with you again."

"I know," I tell him, and I really do.

He softly brushes his lips over mine, making me sigh with happiness.

"So, you were about to tell me something before we were interrupted," he says, pulling away from my lips.

"Oh, yeah." I take a brief pause, gathering the courage I rallied up earlier before Marcel came in.

"Well . . ." I nervously lick my lips. "I was thinking that Gigi and I could move into the house with you."

"Really?" His eyes light up.

"Really."

"When?"

"Well . . . I need to talk to Aunt Elle, give her time to get used to the idea. I don't want to just up and leave her after everything she's done for me and Gigi. But it'll definitely have to be within nine months, as she doesn't have an extra bedroom."

"Nine months?" He frowns. "I was thinking more like nine days."

Seriously?

I stare at him, and he's definitely not getting it.

"Did you get hit harder than I first thought?"

"You're hilarious. But why nine months? And what does Elle not having another bedroom have to do with—oh."

Ding, ding, ding, and he gets it.

He's staring at me, and my heart is in my stomach.

I know Zeus said he wanted more kids with me, but that was when he was trying to win me back. We haven't talked about it since. And we've not been back together very long.

His eyes go down to my stomach. Then, back to my face. "You're pregnant?" he whispers.

"Uh-huh." I nod, nervously chewing my lip.

"With a baby?"

"I hope so because I'm not so keen on the idea of birthing an elephant."

"Hysterical."

"I know."

"You're really pregnant, Dove?"

"I'm really pregnant, Zeus."

His eyes are fixed on me, but I don't know what he's thinking or if he's happy, but I feel the need to tell him, "I was taking the pill. I didn't miss one. Same as when I got pregnant with Gigi. I don't know how it happened. How it keeps happening."

"I don't care how it happened. Just that it did."

"You're happy about this?"

"Dove, I'm fucking ecstatic."

He takes my face in his hands, and he kisses me.

"We're having a baby," he murmurs, his forehead pressed to mine.

"We're having a baby," I echo in confirmation.

"And I have super sperm."

Laughter bubbles up my throat and out of me, relief and happiness filling my chest.

I tip my head back. Staring into his eyes, I give him a look. "Super sperm?"

"I impregnated you twice while you were on the pill. I'm a god."

"Oh Jesus," I complain.

"Nope. Zeus, the God of Thunder, with sperm like lightning."

He grins boyishly, and laughter bursts out of me.

Zeus chuckles, and the sound comes from deep within his chest.

"I'm never going to hear the end of this, am I?" I pseudo-groan, rolling my eyes.

"Nope." He grins and slides his arms around my waist, pulling me even closer, his nose pressed to mine. "Not while I'm around. And I plan on being around for a fuck of a long time, Dove."

Now *that*, I really like the sound of.

Epilogue

"COME ON, MOMMY! IT'S time!"

I walk—sorry, *waddle* over to where Gigi is with her dad and her aunt and uncles, who were tasked with handing out the Chinese lanterns and a lighter to all the adults present at Gigi's fifth birthday party. This includes the parents of her friends from pre-K, Aunt Elle—or Mom, as I call her nowadays—and surprisingly, Zeus's dad, Brett, who has been sober for three months after entering a rehab program after Zeus told him that I was pregnant. I don't know why me being pregnant kick-started his attempt to get sober, but I'm glad it has, and I pray for Zeus and the rest of his siblings that it sticks this time.

Zeus and I agreed that, as Brett is genuinely trying, he could finally meet Gigi, which he did for the first time a month ago. To say he's completely smitten with her is putting it mildly. She has Grandpa Brett wrapped around one of her pinkie fingers. The other is reserved for Zeus. And Ares, Lo, and Missy.

Also, here at the party is Kaden Scott. He recently

moved here to a new facility. He's living in his own place and going in for outpatient treatment.

Zeus and I talked about it, and him being in Arizona, without anyone there, probably wasn't good for his mental state. So, we looked into treatment centers here and found a great one in New York. We flew down to Arizona one weekend, and I got to finally meet him after talking with him on the phone. We discussed the idea with him, and he was on board.

He's been here for three months, and he's just like another member of the family. The great news is that he hasn't been relying on his wheelchair as much, and he has been getting around on crutches.

So, everyone who matters to us is here.

And my baby has turned five. I'm six months pregnant, and I'm totally not crying.

Okay, maybe I'm crying a bit. But these damn pregnancy hormones have got me all topsy-turvy. Even more so since I found out that we're having another girl, so Gigi gets to have a sister. I never had a sister, but I always really wanted one . . . and here I go again with the waterworks.

I press my fingers under my eyes, stopping the emotion.

"You okay, babe?" Zeus quietly asks me as I near him.

"Yep. Just hormones setting me off, like usual."

He grins at me, that smile tugging on my heart, making me want to start blubbering again. He reaches out and grabs my hand, tugging me to him, softly kissing me on the lips.

"Love you," he says low.

"Love you, too."

"Okay, enough with the PDA," Lo complains. "It's grossing me out."

"They kisses alls the time, Uncle Lo," Gigi tells him, giggling.

Lo picks Gigi up, setting her on his hip. "I feel your pain, kid. I had to put up with seeing them kiss all the time when I was a teenager."

"He's just jealous, Gigi girl, because no one wants to date him," Missy teases him.

"No one wants to date you, Uncle Lo?" Gigi looks genuinely concerned for her uncle.

"Everyone wants to date me," Lo assures Gigi, tossing a glare in Missy's direction, who just laughs at him. "Just ask Ares how much puss—"

"Lo . . ." Zeus warns.

"What's puss?" Gigi harps.

"Puss is another word for cats," Ares jumps in, taking Gigi from Lo and setting her up on one of his shoulders, holding her there with his arm.

Sorry, Lo mouths to me.

I smile, telling him it's fine.

"Uncle Lo's getting a kitty?" Gigi's face lights up.

"That's the only puss he'll be getting," Missy quips in a low voice.

I snigger.

Lo gives her a dirty look. "Ares, tell our sister how many phone numbers I got last night."

"He did get a lot," Ares tells Missy.

Lo gives Missy a see-I-told-you-so look.

"You called any of them yet?" she asks.

"No." He gives her an appalled look. "I don't wanna look desperate."

"The only thing you'll look desperate for is a pizza or a cab when you start calling all those fake numbers you were given."

Laughter bursts out of me. I told you, my hormones are all over the place.

The look on Lo's face has me laughing more. It's a mixture of annoyance with a flicker of, *Shit, is she right?*

"Totally gonna go check those numbers now, aren't ya?" Missy prods, winding him up.

"You're a . . ." Lo pauses, searching for what I'm guessing is a kid-friendly comeback. "Female dog."

"Female dog!" Missy laughs, and so do I.

God, I love these guys.

"Okay, enough, children." Zeus takes Gigi from Ares and sets her up on his shoulders. "Can we stop talking about Lo's dating life in front of my impressionable daughter? And get these lanterns lit before dusk is gone."

There's this weird hush between them, and then they all jump to attention with a chorus of . . .

"Yeah, of course!"

"Okay, let's get moving!"

"Everyone, move to the pier!"

As I hold Zeus's hand, we walk down the pier, Gigi still up on his shoulders. With everyone following behind us, we stop at the head of the pier.

Zeus lights a lantern with his lighter and hands it to me. Then, he lights his own.

"Is everyone ready?" Zeus asks.

And we hear a chorus of, "Yes."

"Let me hold, Daddy," Gigi says, making grabby hands.

"Be careful, Gigi girl. They can burn you."

"I've got her," Zeus reassures me.

"Don't forget to make your wish when you let it go," I tell her.

She grins this gorgeous cheeky smile, like she already knows what to wish for.

"Okay, so count of three," Zeus says loudly. "Then, let your lanterns go. Three," Zeus begins. "Two . . . one."

I release my lantern and watch as it starts to make its flight over the water, rising higher, along with everyone else's lanterns.

Then, I briefly close my eyes, just relishing the happiness I feel right now. I can't believe I'm here with Zeus, and I'm pregnant with our second baby.

If you'd said to me a year ago that I'd be here with him, I'd have told you that an asteroid hitting Earth would be more likely.

I hear the gentle sound of Rihanna singing "Umbrella" coming from somewhere behind me, and then the noise of hushed gasps all around has my eyes opening and my head turning.

Zeus is down on his knees beside me.

No. Not knees.

Knee.

Holy crap.

My body slowly turns to him, my eyes not moving from his.

"What are you doing?" I ask.

"Proposing," he says simply.

"I gots the *wing*, Mommy!" Gigi giggles from beside him, holding out a ring box.

"Zeus . . ." Tears fill my eyes.

"You're the love of my life, Dove. It's always been you. From the first moment I saw you at the fair, I was a goner. I fell in love with you then. I love you now. I will go to my grave, loving you. I want you to marry me."

"The *wing* is *weally pwetty*, Mommy!" Gigi thrusts the box at me, and I take it from her.

Fingers trembling, I open the box to see the most beautiful ring I've ever seen. It's a rose gold, diamond-encrusted band, with a large round diamond encircled by smaller diamonds.

My eyes flick to Zeus, a gasp escaping me.

"It was my mother's," he tells me. "It might not fit, but we can have it resized."

Okay, well, now, I'm crying.

I wipe the tears from my face with my hand.

"So, what do you say, Dove? Will you marry me?"

"Says yes, Mommy, 'cause I *weally*, *weally* wanna be a bridesmaid!" Gigi comes to me, wrapping her arms around my leg, hugging me.

My hand goes to her head, holding her close, as tears clog my throat.

I stare down at Zeus, the ring in my hand.

This man . . . he ruins me. Every word. Every look. Every touch.

But there's no one I'd rather be ruined by than him.

Standing here, surrounded by everyone who matters, on my daughter's birthday with our song playing and pretty lanterns lighting up the sky, I give Zeus and Gigi the answer they have been waiting for.

"I say . . . that Gigi is going to make one heck of a beautiful bridesmaid."

Zeus's face cracks into that stunning smile of his.

"Yay!" Gigi squeals.

"Was that a yes?" Lo asks, sounding confused.

"It was a yes," I tell him, my eyes still fixed on Zeus as he rises to his feet. Taking the ring from me, he slips it onto my finger. "A definite, one hundred percent, yes."

Acknowledgments

AS ALWAYS THE BIGGEST thank you goes to my husband and children, who put up with my absences, without complaint (well, mostly without complaint . . . Bella, I'm looking at you!) while I spend time with my imaginary characters, building these crazy, fantastic worlds.

My editor Jovana – I have the best editor ever. You make my life a million times easy. And you put up with me dropping last-minute things on you, constant delays on delivery and extended deadlines, and you never tell me off. You're a saint!

Najla Qamber – my cover designer. I swear, this is our hottest cover yet!

Lauren Abramo – you continue to bring amazing things to the table. If it wasn't for you, I wouldn't be seeing my books in store in my home country, or in other countries around the world. You helped make my dream come true.

My Wether Girls – I flipping love you girls! The best

thing I ever did was setting that group up. It's my safe place.

As always, thank you to each and every member of the blogging world, who work tirelessly to help promote our books, without ask or complaint. We authors couldn't do it without you.

And lastly, to you, the reader, you're the reason I get to live my dream. Thank you.

HEADLINE
ETERNAL